Chinese Medicinal Teas

Simple, Proven, Folk Formulas for Common Diseases & Promoting Health

Zong Xiao-fan & Gary Liscum

BLUE POPPY PRESS, INC.
Boulder, Colorado

Published by:

BLUE POPPY PRESS
A Division of Blue Poppy Enterprises, Inc.
3450 Penrose Place, Suite 110
BOULDER, CO 80301

First Edition, June, 1996
Second Printing, March, 1999

ISBN 0-936185-76-7 LC# 96-85056

COMP Designation: Original work using a standard translational terminology

Printed at Hignell Printing, Ltd. Winnipeg, Canada

10 9 8 7 6 5 4 3 2

Dedication

To our loving sons
Anson and Andi,
who are our best medicinals

XFZ and GAL

Contents

Introduction

Traditional Chinese Medicine, or TCM as it is known in the West, is a rising star in the realm of alternative and complementary health care in the West. In the United States, for instance, over half of all the states have legalized the professional practice of acupuncture and Chinese medicine and there are currently over 50 schools teaching acupuncture and Chinese medicine in the US. Likewise in Europe, Chinese medicine is increasingly being practiced by both non-M.D.'s and M.D.'s alike with schools of acupuncture and Chinese medicine springing up in every country in Western Europe.

When most Westerners think of Chinese medicine, they typically think of acupuncture since it was the first modality of Chinese medicine to receive popular exposure in the media. However, in China, acupuncture is actually not the main modality of TCM. In China, Chinese medicine first and mostly means the prescription of Chinese "herbal" remedies. We say herbal in quotes because, in actuality, Chinese medicine makes use of ingredients from all three kingdoms—animal, vegetable, and mineral. Thus Chinese herbal medicine is a bit of a misnomer since not all the ingredients a Chinese doctor prescribes are, in fact, herbs in the strict sense of this word.

In any case, when a Chinese doctor prescribes an "herbal" remedy, it is usually in the form of a polypharmacy formula administered as a decoction. Poly-pharmacy means administering multiple ingredients at the same time. In the overwhelming majority of cases, Chinese doctors administer formulas consisting of from six to 20 ingredients. Most of these ingredients are roots and rhizomes, root barks, and woody twigs, with a lesser number being leaves, flowers, seeds, fruits, and other ingredients. When such polypharmacy formulas are used, they are typically boiled in water for at least 30 minutes and often for more than an hour. The resulting medicinal liquid is then poured off and is called a *tang* or, literally, a soup. However, when referring to medicinal soups, we usually call these in English a decoction.

Such multiple ingredient soups or decoctions are very strong medicine, and Chinese doctors go to school from four to six years to learn how to prescribe these without negative side effects. After all, if something is strong enough to cure disease in the right person, they must also be strong enough to make someone ill when they are prescribed erroneously. There is no such thing as a universal panacea among medicinal substances. Thus, the prescription of polypharmacy Chinese medicinal decoctions is a professional system of health care requiring lengthy professional training and clinical experience.

Tea as opposed to decoctions

In China, however, there is also a folk tradition of Chinese herbal medicine. Typically, Chinese folk healers use much simpler formulas, often consisting of only one, two, or three ingredients. Often these ingredients are common foods or very common, locally available plants. It is said in Chinese, "Food and medicine share a common source." Further, these folk remedies are often made as infusions instead of more concentrated decoctions. An infusion means that a medicinal ingredient is merely steeped in boiling water for some time rather than being boiled in water as with a decoction.

This book is a collection of such simple Chinese medicinal teas. Some of these are folk formulas and some are recorded in various Chinese books on either herbal medicine or dietary therapy. The majority of the ingredients needed to make such herbal teas are typically available at Western groceries in large cities, at Oriental specialty food stores, and at Western health food stores. Many of the ingredients, such as peach and apricot kernels or dandelion roots may be in your backyard. There is also a chapter in the back of this book with addresses and phone and fax numbers for Chinese medicinal suppliers who sell Chinese medicinals by mail. Thus, the great majority of the ingredients in the formulas in this book are available in the West.

How Chinese medicine works

Chinese medicine treats disease by trying to restore balance to the body. In TCM, all disease is seen as imbalance. Over 2,000 years ago, the authors of the

Nei Jing (Inner Classic), the premier classic of Chinese medicine, stated that if something is vacuous or too little, it should be supplemented; if something is replete or too much, it should be drained; if something is too dry, it should be moistened; if too wet, it should be dried; if too hot, it should be cooled; and if something is too cold, it should be warmed.

In the West, we tend to administer treatments based on a disease diagnosis. In other words, such and such a medicine is good for headache or stomachache. In China, specific medicinal substances are also known to be effective for certain symptoms or diseases. However, most practitioners, whether folk healers or professional practitioners, take their diagnosis a step farther. After all, not every person with a headache has the same bodily constitution. Some people are fat and some are skinny; some are strong and others are weak; some are old and others are young or in the prime of life. Not every person with a headache has the same type of pain in the same location. The pain can be pounding and severe, stabbing and sharp, or dull and low-grade but continuous. The pain can be felt on the top of the head, in the forehead or temples, in the back of the head and neck, like a tight band around the head, on only one side or the other, or all over the head at the same time. Thus it is easy to see that not every headache is the same; nor is every person with pain in the head the same. Each person has their own particular pattern of imbalance.

Therefore, the thing that makes Traditional Chinese Medicine so effective and so safe is that it prescribes both on the basis of the disease or major complaint but also, and even more importantly, on the individual patient's pattern of imbalance or disharmony. This means that two patients with the same Western disease may receive completely different treatments *if their* TCM *patterns are different*. Conversely, two patients with different diseases may receive essentially the same treatment *if their* TCM *pattern is the same*. Because healers in China base their treatment on the individual's pattern, they are prescribing to the whole person, not just their disease or the part or piece that is suffering. It is this treatment based on pattern discrimination that makes Chinese medicine the holistic, safe, and effective medicine it is. Further, the main difference between the Chinese folk herbalist and the professional practitioner

3

of TCM is the latter's extensive training and increased ability to accurately discriminate patients' patterns of imbalance and prescribe the right medicine for the right pattern.

Who should use this book

This book is meant for both lay readers interested in Chinese herbal medicine and professional TCM practitioners alike. Professionally trained practitioners of acupuncture who already know how to do a TCM pattern discrimination will find these very simple remedies an easy way to begin incorporating Chinese herbal medicine into their practice. The ingredients are relatively cheap, easily available, and, compared to stronger medicinals which require prolonged decoction or to larger, more complex, polypharmacy formulas, are generally safer to use with a lesser degree of knowledge. These formulas are also useful in areas where the full range of Chinese medicinals is not easily accessible. Thus, this book can serve as a sort of emergency formulary or as a formulary for areas where Chinese medicinals are hard to get or simply unavailable.

Lay readers attempting to use this manual should take care to match up not only the disease indications, such as headache or vomiting, but also the other symptoms which go along with the TCM pattern for which each formula is indicated. In many cases, we have included the most important differentiating signs and symptoms of these patterns in order to help select the right formula for the right pattern of disease. Those not already trained in TCM pattern discrimination should see the bibliography at the end of this book. There is both a bibliography of our Chinese language sources and an English language bibliography of books about Chinese medicine. Further information on TCM pattern discrimination can be found in a number of these English language books, most notably Ted Kaptchuk's *The Web That Has No Weaver: Understanding Chinese Medicine*.

For those lay readers with serious complaints, such as various types of cancers as found in Chapter 13, neither the authors nor the publishers recommend or endorse self-treatment by laypersons. Therefore, lay readers wishing to make use of the tea formulas given in this book for more serious diseases should first

4

seek a TCM pattern discrimination by a qualified professional practitioner of TCM and then should follow that practitioner's recommendations about specific formulas appearing in this book. At the end of this book, the reader will also find the names and addresses of several professional associations which will help make finding such a local professional practitioner, at least in the United States, easier.

Medicinal identifications

The ingredients in this book have been identified in three ways. These are 1) by common English name, 2) by Latinate pharmacological identification, and 3) by Pinyin in that order. Pinyin is the system of writing Chinese words in the Roman alphabet which is the standard method of romanization used in the People's Republic of China. If the medicinal is a common ingredient found in food stores or growing either cultivated or wild in the West, we have first given its common English name. If this ingredient is also a medicinal sold by Chinese herb suppliers, then its Latin name is also given, followed by its Pinyin name in parentheses. If a medicinal is not commonly found in the West but must be ordered from a Chinese herb supplier, only its Latin and Pinyin names are given. It should be noted that the Pinyin names approximate the pronunciation of the Chinese name in what was known as Mandarin and is now know as Common Speech (*Pu Tung Hua*). We say approximate pronunciation because this system of romanization was created in the 1950's for Russian speakers, not English speakers. Therefore, Westerners trying to pronounce these names in Chinese from the Pinyin spelling are rarely understood by native speakers. This problem is compounded by the fact that many, if not most, Chinese herb suppliers are Cantonese or Vietnamese Chinese who may not speak Mandarin in any case.

Uncooked vs. Fresh

In some cases, medicinal herbs are preceded by the words fresh (*xian*) or uncooked (*sheng*). Uncooked is a technical term in TCM herbal medicine. It means that the ingredient has not undergone any previous processing using fire. When the word uncooked is used, it is to differentiate the unprocessed version of the ingredients rather than a version which has undergone some previous cooking procedure. The word uncooked typically precedes the names of herbal medicinals which are commonly used in their uncooked state and also in some processed form, such as stir-fried or mix-fried. In these cases, the reader knows that it is the uncooked form and not one of the various processed forms of the medicinal that is wanted. For instance, if a formula calls for uncooked Licorice, *i.e.*, uncooked Radix Glycyrrhizae (*Sheng Gan Cao*), then the reader also knows that the purpose of the Licorice is, at least in part, to clear heat and resolve toxins as opposed to supplementing the heart and spleen. If one wants to supplement the heart and spleen using Licorice, then it is the mix-fried version one wants to use. Fresh means that it is the freshly picked, undried plant that is to be used. In the overwhelming majority of cases, the uncooked version of a Chinese herb will not be freshly picked but will be dried. However, in the case of uncooked Rhizoma Zingiberis (*Sheng Jiang*), the uncooked form of Ginger is also fresh Ginger.

How to make an infusion

Although each formula does include its own instructions for preparation, one may say something about making a Chinese herbal infusion or tea in general. In its simplest form, the ingredients are placed directly into a container. Boiling water is then poured over these ingredients, the contents are stirred so that all the surfaces of the ingredients come into contact with the boiling water, and a lid is then placed on top of the container's mouth. Putting a lid on the container helps maintain the temperature, usually 80-95°F. It also helps insure that volatile, aromatic medicinal substances are not lost through evaporation. The medicinals are then allowed to steep or infuse for 10-30 minutes. For medicinals which require a longer infusion time, a thermos bottle or thermos cup is useful to help maintain the proper temperature. When the time is right, the ingredients are then strained out of the infusion and the medicinal tea is drunk or saved for later use.

Usually, dried herbs are powdered, coarsely ground, sliced, or broken into pieces, while fresh herbs are likewise sliced or torn apart in order to expand their surface area. This facilitates the extraction of their active ingredients. This

6

is especially important when ingredients are simply infused rather than decocted. Often, these ingredients can be used more than once. That means they can be reinfused by pouring fresh boiling water over them one or more times after their initial use. Thus one can extract their full medicinal benefit.

How to take a Chinese medicinal tea

Most Chinese herbal teas are drunk warm or hot unless specified otherwise, and it is also best if the tea is drunk the same day as it is made. The dosages given in this book are for one packet or *bao*, and one *bao* typically equals one day's dose. Thus the medicinals in one packet can be steeped over and over throughout the day. This is especially important for conditions which do best when a constant level of medicine should be maintained in the body continuously. In places where it says that the formula can be drunk as a tea, this means that it can and should be drunk repeatedly throughout the day as a beverage. As to amount per dose, one should follow the guidelines in the text under each formula.

When to take Chinese medicinal teas

There are also a few rules on the proper time to take Chinese medicinal teas. Formulas that promote perspiration and resolve the exterior should be taken warm. The body should be kept covered and treatment should be stopped once perspiration appears on the body. Supplementing and boosting formulas should be taken before meals in order to facilitate their complete absorption. Formulas for gastrointestinal complaints should be taken after meals in order to help with the actual process of digestion. Calming or sedative formulas are best taken before sleep. Formulas that are designed to treat the throat should be swallowed slowly in order to moisten the throat and achieve maximum effect. Teas for treating the urological system should be taken repeatedly and continuously in order to maintain a constant solution in the urine. This also helps dilute the urine, clear the urinary tract, and benefit the expulsion of turbidity and dampness. Teas taken for the prevention of epidemic toxins, such as measles, diphtheria, and infectious hepatitis, should be taken in their appropriate season. And teas for promoting longevity or for the treatment of chronic diseases need to be taken on a regular and long-term basis.

The advantages of infusions over decoctions

One advantage to an infusion as opposed to a decoction is that it preserves the volatile oils and aromatic medicinal substances that are lost when certain ingredients are boiled. For instance, Mint (Herba Menthae Haplocalycis [*Bo He*]), Chrysanthemum flowers (Flos Chrysanthemi Morifolii [*Ju Hua*]), and Senna leaves (Folium Sennae [*Fan Xie Ye*]) lose their medicinal strength if decocted and should only be infused or decocted for a very short period of time. Other substances which should not be boiled are the various gelatins, such as Gelatinum Corii Asini (*E Jiao*), Gelatinum Plastri Testudinis (*Gui Ban Jiao*), and Gelatinum Cornu Cervi (*Lu Jiao Jiao*). These should only be allowed to dissolve in boiling water.

Secondly, patient compliance is typically higher with infusions than decoctions. Chinese herbal decoctions are notoriously bitter. There is even a saying in Chinese which goes to the effect that, "The bitterer the brew, the better the medicine." Although that may be the case, medicine is useless if the patient refuses to drink it. Infusions are usually much milder in taste than decoctions and, therefore, patients often will drink them more readily. Another consideration is that infusions are quicker to prepare. A decoction may take anywhere from 30 minutes to more than an hour to cook, whereas an infusion is done as quickly as water can be brought to a boil and then the medicinals simply steeped. During this short steeping period, the patient can also do something else without having to worry about their herbs either boiling away or boiling over. Thus the relative ease of preparing infusions also makes them suitable for fast-paced, busy modern Westerners.

The drawbacks are that not every Chinese medicinal ingredient lends itself to infusion. Many of the ingredients of Chinese medicine simply require decoction before their active ingredients become available. That being said, there are still lots and lots of ingredients which can be used as infusions just as they are, while powdering other ingredients makes them also infusible as well.

Chinese medicinal teas & diet

As stated above, Chinese medicinal teas are an excellent treatment choice when a full Chinese pharmacy is unavailable, when they are used as an adjunct to acupuncture and moxibustion, for first aid, or as an introduction to Chinese herbal medicine for beginning practitioners or new patients. However, for Chinese medicinal teas to get their full effect, it is very important that the person's diet also be adjusted according to the principles of Chinese dietary therapy. Since many, if not most, chronic diseases are caused and perpetuated at least in part by faulty diet, it is very important that the Chinese medicinal teas described in this book be supported by the right diet.

What a right diet is for any particular individual is based, just as the herbal teas described in this book, on their TCM pattern of disharmony. In general, TCM practitioners recommend what is called a "clear, bland diet." This means a mostly, though not exclusively, vegetarian diet high in complex carbohydrates from grains and beans, and high in vegetables and fruit. In the clear, bland diet of Chinese medicine, foods like meats, sugars, fats, oils, salt, and spices are all used sparingly as condiments rather than as everyday main dishes. Beyond this clear, bland diet, however, each individual should eat those foods which help them maintain their own personal healthy balance and equilibrium. That means that some people should eat more meat and others less. Some people should eat more warming spices and others should avoid these. Some people should drink some alcohol and others should abstain completely.

Exactly what your optimum Chinese medical diet is can only be determined by a professional diagnosis by a trained and qualified, professional TCM practitioner. Such a practitioner can do a TCM pattern discrimination and tell you exactly which foods are good for you and which are not so good or even harmful to your health. If your TCM diet is correct, then the Chinese medicinal teas described in this book will be able to carry you to even greater balance and well-being. If the TCM diet is not correct, taking the teas described in this book will be like bailing on one side as water is swamping your boat from the other. For more information about Chinese dietary therapy, see Bob Flaws' *Arisal of the Clear: A Simple Guide to Healthy Eating According to Traditional Chinese Medicine,* as well as his *The Book of Jook: Chinese Medicinal Porridges, a Healthy Alternative to the Typical Western Breakfast* and *Chinese Medicinal Wines & Elixirs,* all published by Blue Poppy Press.

About *Camellia Thea*

One of the most common ingredients in the formulas contained in this book is Folium Camelliae Theae (*Cha Ye*). This refers to the leaves of the tea bush from which we get the tea we use as a daily beverage—as in, "Would you prefer tea or coffee?" (From here on, where tea refers to an infusion of this particular plant, we have capitalized the word, *e.g.,* Tea, to distinguish it from tea meaning an infusion as opposed to a decoction.) The cultivation and use of this plant in China has a long history. Tea drinking is so much a part of Chinese culture we even have a saying in English, "Not for all the Tea in China." Thus a few words about the use of Tea as both a beverage and as a medicinal substance are in order.

Although some people believe that Tea was introduced from India by Buddhist monks some time in the first millennium, the earliest written mention of Tea in the Chinese literature is found in the *Er Ya (Elegant Poems)* written during the Western Zhou dynasty (1100-771 BCE). It is recorded here that the Chinese people had some knowledge of Tea at that time. In the *Shi Jing (Poetry Classic)*, one of China's earliest collections of poetry, there are also poems about Tea. In the Han dynasty (206 BCE-220 CE), the *Shi Ji (Historical Records)* say that Tea leaves were given as a war tribute by the Bashu tribe of southern China to an imperial expedition.

During the Three Kingdoms (220-265 CE) and the Jin dynasty (265-420 CE), drinking Tea gradually became popular in China. It is said that the last emperor of the Eastern Wu (222-280 CE), Sun Hao, encouraged his ministers to drink liquor to the point of drunkenness at banquets. One minister could not drink alcohol. So the emperor secretly let him substitute Tea for wine. Since that time, Confucian scholars began to entertain guests with Tea and this has been a custom in China ever since.

During the very prosperous Tang dynasty (618-907 CE), commoners, following the custom of the nobility, also began to drink Tea. By the Song Dynasty (960-1297 CE), a famous minister and scholar, Wang An-shi, could write, "The use of Tea is equal to rice and salt; one cannot be without it for a day." At this time, historical records indicate that Tea leaves were picked and then made into Tea cakes. These cakes were baked or roasted to a red color. When a cup of Tea was wanted, a portion of such a cake was broken off and then pounded into a powder. This powder was then placed in a porcelain container. Boiling water was poured over this powder to make an infusion. Chinese even to this day drink and distinguish two basic types of beverage Tea—green Tea (*Lu Cha*) and red, *i.e.*, black Tea (*Hong Cha*). Scallions, ginger, and tangerine peel were also commonly added for flavor. In the Jin or Tatar dynasty (1115-1234 CE), there was the custom of making tea with ginger and cardamon. This custom was probably imported by Buddhist monks from India as this is still how Tea is commonly drunk in India today (along with milk and sugar).

The use of Tea as a medicinal substance in China also has a long history. There are mentions of the medicinal use of Tea in Wang Tao's Tang dynasty *Wai Tai Mi Yao (Secret Essentials of a Frontier Official)*, Wang Huai-yin *et al.*'s Song dynasty *Tai Ping Sheng Hui Fang (Tai Ping Imperial Grace Formulary)*, Hu Si-hui's *Yin Shan Zheng Yao (Correct Essentials of Drinking & Eating)*, and Zhu Ti's Ming dynasty *Pu Ji Fang (Universal Benefit Formulas)*. In Li Shi-zhen's Ming dynasty *Ben Cao Gang Mu (The Detailed Outline of the Materia Medica)*, it is said:

Tea mainly treats dyspnea, rapid [breathing], and cough and it removes phlegm.

Tea is bitter and cold. It is able to downbear fire. Fire produces hundreds of diseases. When fire is downborne, the clear can ascend.

For phlegm dyspnea and cough with inability to lie down, [use] 1 *liang* of good, powdered Tea, and 1 *liang* of Bombyx Batryticatus (*Bai Jiang Can*), powdered. Place in a bowl. Pour in 1 small cup of boiling water. Before lying down [to sleep], add some [water] and drink some more.

By the Qing dynasty (1644-1911), it was common practice to use Tea medicinally at the imperial court. In the *Ci Xi Guang Xu Yi Fang Xuan Yi (A Discussion of the Medical Formulas of Ci Xi & Guang Xu)*, there are 20 medicinal Tea formulas for the Dowager Empress Ci Xi and Emperor Guang Xu.

Formulas such as Harmonize the Spleen Tea (*He Pi Cha*) for Guang Xu and Clear Heat Tea (*Qing Re Cha*) for Ci Xi are examples.

In China today, there is a great deal of interest in the medicinal properties and uses of Tea and much research is being conducted on this ubiquitous beverage. Tea is credited with reducing weight and serum cholesterol to preventing certain types of cancer. Truly, "Food and medicine share a common source."

1
Respiratory Diseases

Common Cold Teas

Colds and flu are very common illnesses and can occur at any time of the year. In Traditional Chinese Medicine (TCM), they are usually divided into two major patterns: wind cold and wind heat. However, other factors involved may include summerheat, dampness, and constitutional deficiencies. Seasonal weather and disease pathogens, therefore, vary as do clinical symptoms. In TCM, it is important to pick the right tea for the right pattern of signs and symptoms.

Ginger & Sugar Tea (*Jiang Tang Cha*)

Uncooked ginger, *i.e.*, uncooked Rhizoma Zingiberis (*Sheng Jiang*)	3 slices
Brown sugar (*Hong Tang*)	Amount to taste

Method of administration: Place the ingredients in a cup and pour in boiling water. Drink warm, 1-2 packets per day at any time of the day.

Functions: Promotes sweating and resolves the exterior, warms the center and harmonizes the stomach

Indications: This tea is suitable for a wind cold exterior pattern with aversion to cold, fever, headache, cough, and no sweating. It may also be used for nausea, vomiting, abdominal distention, and stomach pain since uncooked Ginger not only relieves the exterior but also harmonizes the stomach.

Ginger & Perilla Leaf Tea (*Jiang Su Cha*)

Uncooked ginger, *i.e.,* uncooked Rhizoma Zingiberis (*Sheng Jiang*)   3 grams
Perilla leaf, *i.e.,* Folium Perillae Frutescentis (*Zi Su Ye*)   3 grams

Method of administration: Cut the fresh ginger into tiny threads. Place the perilla leaf and ginger in a cup and pour in boiling water. Let the mixture soak for 10 minutes and then drink the tea warm. Use 1 packet in the morning and 1 in the afternoon.

Functions: Courses wind and scatters cold, rectifies the qi and harmonizes the stomach

Indications: This tea is suitable for wind cold exterior patterns with headache and fever. It is also suitable for nausea, vomiting, stomachache, abdominal distention, and gastrointestinal complaints associated with the common cold. This formula uses herbs in small quantities. It is convenient, practical, and suitable for both the prevention and treatment of disease.

Note: Perilla leaves are also called Beefsteak leaves in English and are available from many seed companies. In Japanese, they are called *Chiso* or *Shiso*.

Perilla & Notopterygium Tea (*Su Qiang Cha*)

Perilla leaf, *i.e.,* Folium Perillae Frutescentis (*Zi Su Ye*)   9 grams
Radix Et Rhizoma Notopterygii (*Qiang Huo*)   9 grams
Tea leaves, *i.e.,* Folium Camilliae Theae (*Cha Ye*)   9 grams

Method of administration: Grind these three ingredients into a coarse powder. Place them in a cup and pour in boiling water. Drink warm, 1 packet per day at any time.

Functions: Resolves the exterior with warm, acrid ingredients, scatters cold and dispels wind

Indications: This tea is suitable for wind cold exterior patterns with aversion to cold, fever, headache, no sweating, and aching pain in the limbs.

Common Cold Tea (*Gan Mao Cha*)

Radix Et Rhizoma Notoptergyii (*Qiang Huo*)	30 grams
Radix Angelicae Dahuricae (*Bai Zhi*)	12 grams
Radix Scutellariae Baicalensis (*Huang Qin*)	15 grams

Method of administration: Place these three ingredients in a container and pour in boiling water. Drink warm, 1 packet per day at any time.

Functions: Dispels wind and scatters cold

Indications: This tea is suitable for wind cold exterior patterns with headache, body pain, nasal congestion, runny nose, aversion to cold, and fever. It is very effective.

Angelica & Schizonepeta Tea (*Bai Zhi Jing Jie Cha*)

Radix Angelicae Dahuricae (*Bai Zhi*)	30 grams
Herba Seu Flos Schizonepetae Tenuifoliae (*Jing Jie*)	3 grams
Tea leaves, *i.e.*, Folium Camelliae Theae (*Cha Ye*)	3 grams

Method of administration: Grind the angelica root and schizonepeta into a fine powder. Prepare the Tea leaves as an infusion with boiling water. Ingest 6 grams of the powdered herbs and then drink the tea. This formula may be taken 2 times per day.

Functions: Dispels wind and scatters cold, resolves the exterior and relieves pain

Indications: This tea is suitable for the initial stage of a wind cold exterior pattern with aversion to cold, fever, nasal congestion, a clear, runny nose, headache, and toothache.

Five Spirits Tea (*Wu Shen Cha*)

Herba Seu Flos Schizonepetae Tenuifoliae (*Jing Jie*)	10 grams
Perilla leaf, *i.e.*, Folium Perillae Frutescentis (*Zi Su Ye*)	10 grams
Uncooked ginger, *i.e.*, uncooked Rhizoma Zingiberis (*Sheng Jiang*)	10 grams
Brown sugar (*Hong Tang*)	30 grams
Tea leaves, *i.e.*, Folium Camelliae Theae (*Cha Ye*)	6 grams

Method of administration: Boil the schizonepeta, perilla leaves, fresh ginger, and Tea over low heat for 15-20 minutes. Then add the brown sugar. Remove from the heat as soon as the brown sugar has dissolved. Use 1 packet per day. This tea may be taken twice daily.

Functions: Dispels wind, scatters cold, and relieves pain

Indications: This tea is suitable for the treatment of wind cold patterns with fear of cold, body pain, and no sweating.

Perilla Leaf Tea (*Zi Su Ye Cha*)

Perilla leaf, *i.e.*, Folium Perillae Frutescentis (*Zi Su Ye*)	16 grams
Brown sugar (*Hong Tang*)	Amount to taste

Method of administration: Dry the herb and grind into a coarse powder. Place the herb into a container, pour in boiling water, and then add the brown sugar. Allow the brown sugar to dissolve. Use 1 packet per day. Drink this freely as a tea.

Functions: Dispels wind and scatters cold

Indications: This tea is suitable for the initial stage of a wind cold pattern with nasal congestion, runny nose, fear of cold, and pain in all the limbs and joints.

Scallion & Sliced Ginger Tea (*Cong Tou Jiang Pian Cha*)

Scallion, *i.e.,* Bulbus Allii Fistulosi (*Cong Tou*)	10 grams
Uncooked ginger, *i.e.*, uncooked Rhizoma Zingiberis (*Sheng Jiang*)	3 grams
Brown sugar (*Hong Tang*)	Amount to taste

Method of administration: Wash the scallion and uncooked ginger well and cut into slices. Place these into a pot with the brown sugar, add water, and boil for 10 minutes. Pour off the resulting liquid and drink while hot. Use 1 packet per day. For best results, after taking this tea, cover up with a blanket to induce a light sweat.

Functions: Promotes sweating and resolves the exterior

Indications: This tea is suitable for externally contracted wind cold patterns with headache, aversion to cold, nasal congestion, and clear nasal mucous.

Mulberry, Chrysanthemum & Fermented Soybean Tea (*Sang Ye Ju Hua Xiang Chi Cha*)

Mulberry leaf, *i.e.*, Folium Mori Albi (*Sang Ye*)	6 grams
Chrysanthemum flower, *i.e.*, Flos Chrysanthemi Morifolii (*Ju Hua*)	6 grams
Unsalted, fermented soybean, *i.e.*, Semen Praeparatus Sojae (*Xiang Chi*)	6 grams
Pear skin, *i.e.*, Cortex Fructi Pyri (*Li Pi*)	6 grams

Method of administration: Place the herbs into a pot, cover with water, and simmer briefly. Discard the dregs and save the liquid. Use 1 packet per day. Drink freely as a tea.

Functions: Clears heat and resolves the exterior, moistens the lungs and checks coughing

Indications: This tea is suitable for a wind heat external pattern with dryness. Its symptoms are fever, slight aversion to wind and chill, headache, some sweating, cough with scanty phlegm, a dry throat and nose, and thirst. Other symptoms are a red tongue with a thin, white or slightly yellow coating and a floating, rapid pulse.

Mulberry, Chrysanthemum, & Lophatherum Tea (*Sang Ju Zhu Ye Cha*)

Mulberry leaf, *i.e.*, Folium Mori Albi (*Sang Ye*)	5 grams
Chrysanthemum flower, *i.e.*, Flos Chrysanthemi Morifolii (*Ju Hua*)	5 grams
Folium Lophatheri Gracilis (*Dan Zhu Ye*)	30 grams
Rhizoma Imperatae Cylindricae (*Bai Mao Gen*)	30 grams
Field mint or peppermint, *i.e.*, Herba Menthae Haplocalycis (*Bo He*)	3 grams
White sugar (*Bai Tang*)	20 grams

Method of administration: Place all these ingredients in a cup, pour in boiling water, and soak for 10 minutes. Alternatively, boil the herbs for 5 minutes, add the sugar, and drink freely as a tea. Use 1 packet per day.

Functions: Clears heat, dispels wind, and resolves the exterior

Indications: This tea is suitable for a wind heat exterior pattern with aversion to cold, fever, headache, body pain, nasal congestion, runny nose, and mild swelling of the cheek although the affected area is not red. Other symptoms include a thin, white tongue coating and a rapid, floating pulse.

Three Flowers Tea (*San Hua Cha*)

Honeysuckle flower, *i.e.*, Flos Lonicerae Japonicae (*Jin Yin Hua*)	15 grams
Chrysanthemum flower, *i.e.*, Flos Chrysanthemi Morifolii (*Ju Hua*)	10 grams

Jasmine flower, *i.e.*, Flos Jasmini (*Mo Li Hua*)   3 grams

Method of administration: Place these three flowers in a teacup, pour in boiling water, and soak for 10-15 minutes. Use 1 packet per day. Drink this freely as a tea.

Functions: Clears heat and resolves toxins

Indications: This tea is suitable for a wind heat exterior pattern with heat toxins as evidenced by a sore, swollen throat, carbuncles and sores. It may also be taken frequently by individuals with exuberant fire, since it has the effect of downbearing fire.

Mulberry, Chrysanthemum & Loquat Tea (*Sang Ju Pi Pa Cha*)

Wild chrysanthemum flower, *i.e.*, Flos Chrysanthemi Indici
   (*Ye Ju Hua*)   10 grams
Mulberry leaf, *i.e.*, Folium Mori Albi (*Sang Ye*)   10 grams
Loquat leaf, *i.e.*, Folium Eriobotryae Japonicae (*Pi Pa Ye*)   10 grams

Method of administration: Grind these herbs into a coarse powder, briefly boil in water, and then pour off the liquid. Use 1 packet per day. This tea may be taken frequently for 3-5 days.

Functions: Clears heat and dispels wind, resolves the exterior and transforms phlegm

Indications: This is suitable for the treatment of flu symptoms exhibiting a wind heat exterior pattern with phlegm. The symptoms are recent onset, fever, slight sweating, sore throat, cough with yellow phlegm, a red tongue with a thin, slightly slimy, yellow tongue coating, and a floating, slippery, wiry. rapid pulse.

Flu Tea (*Liu Gan Cha*)

Rhizoma Guanzhong (*Guan Zhong*)	30 grams
Radix Isatidis Seu Baphicacanthi (*Ban Lan Gen*)	30 grams
Licorice root, *i.e.*, Radix Glycyrrhizae Uralensis (*Gan Cao*)	15 grams

Method of administration: Place these herbs in a cup and pour in boiling water. Use 1 packet per day. Drink this freely as a tea at any time.

Functions: Clears heat and resolves toxins, dispels wind and disinhibits the throat

Indications: This tea is a suitable formula for flu with pronounced sore throat exhibiting a wind heat pattern with heat toxins. It may also be used preventively. These herbs all have relatively strong effect against flu viruses.

Elsholtzia Tea (*Xiang Ru Cha*)

Herba Elsholtziae Splendentis (*Xiang Ru*)	10 grams
Cortex Magnoliae Officinalis (*Hou Po*)	5 grams
Hyacinth bean, *i.e.*, Semen Dolicohoris Lablab (*Bai Bian Dou*)	5 grams

Method of administration: Use scissors to cut the cleaned elsholtzia and magnolia bark into pieces. Stir-fry the hyacinth beans until they are cooked and then pound into pieces. Place the herbs into a thermos and pour in boiling water. Seal tightly and let the herbs soak for 1 hour. Use 1 packet per day. Drink this freely as a tea.

Functions: Dispels summerheat and resolves the exterior, harmonizes the center and transforms dampness

Indications: This is suitable for the treatment of summertime colds and flus with fever, headache, heaviness of the head, chest oppression, fatigue, abdominal pain, vomiting, and diarrhea.

Codonopsis & Perilla Leaf Tea (*Shen Su Cha*)

Radix Codonopsitis Pilosulae (*Dang Shen*)   15 grams
Perilla leaf, *i.e.*, Folium Perillae Frutescentis (*Zi Su Ye*)   12 grams

Method of administration: Place the herbs in a teapot, pour in boiling water, and let soak. Drink 1 packet per day.

Functions: Boosts the qi at the same time as it resolves the exterior

Indications: This tea is suitable for the treatment of an exterior wind cold pattern in persons with a concomitant qi vacuity. It is also a relatively good preventive tea for older and weak individuals during the flu season.

Preventing the Common Cold Tea (*Yu Fang Gan Mao Cha*)

Radix Isatidis Seu Baphicacanthi (*Ban Lan Gen*)   50 grams
Folium Daqingye (*Da Qing Ye*)   50 grams
Wild chrysanthemum flower, *i.e.,* Flos Chrysanthem Indici
    (*Ye Ju Hua*)   30 grams
Honeysuckle flower, *i.e.,* Flos Lonicerae Japonicae (*Jin Yin Hua*) 30 grams

Method of administration: Place the herbs in a large cup and pour in boiling water. Let them soak for a short time and then drink the liquid. Use 1 packet per day. Drink this freely as a tea.

Functions: Clears heat and resolves toxins

Indications: This tea is suitable as a preventative for flu. It may also be used as a preventative for epidemic meningitis, epidemic hepatitis, and epidemic infection of the respiratory tract, especially viral infections.

Bronchitis Tea Formulas

Bronchitis means the acute or chronic inflammation of the membranes of the bronchial mucosa. This inflammation may be caused by either a bacterial or viral infection, or it may be due to chronic irritation by physical or chemical factors. Its main symptoms are cough and expectoration of phlegm. In TCM, acute bronchitis is usually due to externally contracted repletions. If improperly treated, this condition may occur repeatedly and this may eventually damage the viscera. If this occurs, it is called an internal damage cough. Other causes of chronic bronchitis may be weak spleen function that leads to damp and phlegm accumulation in the lungs, while other patterns may involve the kidneys. Thus the patterns and symptoms of this disease are variable and the appropriate herbal tea should be given according to each individual's condition.

Tangerine Peel Tea (*Ju Hong Cha*)

Tangerine peel, *i.e.*, Pericarpium Citri Erythrocarpae (*Ju Hong*)   3-6 grams
Green tea, *i.e.*, Folium Camelliae Theae (*Lu Cha*)   4.5 grams

Method of administration: Place the two ingredients in a cup, pour in boiling water, and let soak. Then place the cup in a covered pot filled with water to halfway up the cup. Steam the herbs in this covered pot for 20 minutes. Use 1 packet per day. Drink this freely as a tea.

Functions: Moistens the lungs and transforms phlegm, rectifies the qi and checks cough

Indications: This tea is suitable for the treatment of cough with profuse, white phlegm or sticky, tenacious phlegm which is difficult to expectorate.

Radish Tea (*Luo Bo Cha*)

White radish, *i.e.*, Radix Raphani Sativi (*Bai Luo Bo*)   100 grams
Tea leaves, *i.e.*, Folium Camelliae Theae (*Cha Ye*)   5 grams

Salt (*Yan*)   Amount to taste

Note: Radish here refers to the large, white radish called *Daikon* in Japanese and sold at most large grocery or Oriental specialty food stores.

Method of administration: Pour boiling water over the Tea, soak for 5 minutes, and reserve the liquid. Wash the radish well, slice, then cook thoroughly, seasoning with salt. Place the radish in a cup and pour in the tea water. Use 2 packets per day. Drink warm at any time.

Functions: Clears heat and transforms phlegm, rectifies the qi and increases the appetite

Indications: This tea is suitable for cough with profuse phlegm and no thought for eating food. It is most appropriate for individuals with excessive phlegm and cough caused by lung heat.

Mint & Licorice Tea (*Bo He Gan Cao Cha*)

Field mint or peppermint, *i.e.*, Herba Menthae Haplocalycis (*Bo He*)   9 grams
Fresh licorice root, *i.e.*, uncooked Radix Glycyrrhizae Uralensis
    (*Sheng Gan Cao*)   3 grams
White sugar (*Bai Tang*)   Amount to taste

Method of administration: Place the licorice root in a pot and add 500ml of water. Decoct for 10 minutes; then add the mint. Briefly decoct again and strain off the liquid. Add sugar and stir well. Drink when cool.

Functions: Clears the lungs and stops cough, resolves toxins and disinhibits the throat

Indications: This tea is suitable for the treatment of cough due to a wind heat exterior pattern with sore, itching throat and a hoarse voice.

Note: Do *not* substitute spearmint instead of common field or peppermint. It is warming and this tea is meant to clear heat with cool ingredients. Likewise, white sugar is cooling, while brown sugar is warming.

Engender Liquids & Harmonize the Stomach Tea (*Sheng Jin He Wei Cha*)

Large pears, *i.e.*, Fructus Pyri Communis (*Da Li*)	3 fruits
Nodus Nelumbinis Nuciferae (*Ou Jie*)	1 piece
Ramulus Nelumbinis Nuciferae (*He Geng*)	1 piece
Fasciculis Vascularis Citri Reticulatae (*Ju Luo*)	3 grams
Plumula Nelumbinis Nuciferae (*Lian Xin*)	10 pieces
Licorice root, *i.e.*, Radix Glycyrrhizae Uralensis (*Gan Cao*)	3 grams
Uncooked Ginger, *i.e.*, uncooked Rhizoma Zingiberis (*Sheng Jiang*)	3 slices
Ginseng, *i.e.*, Radix Panacis Ginseng (*Ren Shen*)	6 grams

Method of administration: Peel the pears, the lotus node, and the fresh ginger and then pound into a liquid. Next, chop the lotus stem into pieces, slice the ginseng, and place these together in a pot with the tangerine pith, licorice root, and lotus plumules. Add water and boil for 30 minutes. Let cool; then strain off the liquid. Mix the two liquids together, stirring evenly. Use 1 packet per day. Drink this freely as a tea.

Functions: Moistens the lungs, engenders liquids, and stops cough

Indications: This tea is suitable for coughs caused by lung dryness or a dry throat caused by stomach dryness damaging liquids with stomach reflux and hiccoughs.

Biota Twig Tea (*Ce Bai Cha Ye*)

Cacumen Biotae Orientalis (*Ce Bai Ye*)	6 grams

Method of administration: Loosely break up the biota twigs, place them in a pot, and boil briefly in water. Strain off the liquid and drink. Use 1 packet per day.

Functions: Cools the blood, stops bleeding, and settles cough

Indications: This tea is suitable for the treatment of lung heat with cough, expectoration of blood, or blood-streaked mucus.

Coltsfoot Flower Tea (*Dong Hua Cha*)

Tea leaves, *i.e.*, Folium Camelliae Theae (*Cha Ye*)	6 grams
Coltsfoot flower, *i.e.*, Flos Tussilaginis Farfarae (*Kuan Dong Hua*)	3 grams
Radix Asteris Tatarici (*Zi Wan*)	3 grams

Method of administration: Place the above three ingredients in a cup, pour in boiling water, and soak. Use 1 packet per day. Drink this freely as a tea.

Functions: Dispels phlegm, stops cough, and calms dyspnea

Indications: This tea is suitable for the treatment of bronchitis and asthma.

Note: Japanese research suggests that coltsfoot should only be taken for relatively short periods of time.

Tangerine Tea (*Ju Cha*)

Tea leaves, *i.e.*, Folium Camelliae Theae (*Cha Ye*)	2 grams
Dry tangerine peel, *i.e.*, Pericarpium Citri Reticulatae (*Gan Ju Pi*)	2 grams

Method of administration: Place these two ingredients in a cup, pour in boiling water, and steep for 10 minutes.

Functions: Stops cough and transforms phlegm, rectifies the qi and harmonizes the stomach

Indications: This tea is suitable for chronic bronchitis, profuse phlegm, and gastric discomfort. This formula is only for mild conditions, not serious ones.

Fritillaria & Radish Tea (*Chuan Bei Lai Fu Cha*)

Bulbus Fritillariae Cirrhosae (*Chuan Bei Mu*)	15 grams
Radish seeds, *i.e.,* Semen Raphani Sativi (*Lai Fu Zi*)	15 grams

Method of administration: Grind these two herbs into a coarse powder. Place this powder in a cup, pour in boiling water, and let soak. It may also be boiled. Use 1 packet per day. Drink it freely as a tea.

Functions: Moistens the lungs and transforms phlegm, downbears counterflow, stops cough, and calms dyspnea

Indications: This tea is suitable for the treatment of chronic bronchitis with cough and profuse phlegm.

Honey & Egg Tea (*Mi Dan Cha*)

Honey (*Feng Mi*)	35 grams
Chicken egg (*Ji Dan*)	1 egg

Method of administration: Place the honey in a pot, add water, and bring to a boil. Crack the egg and beat evenly. Pour the boiled honey water into the egg bowl. Drink warm, 1-2 doses per day.

Functions: Diffuses the lungs, moistens the throat, and stops cough

Indications: This tea is suitable for chronic bronchitis and a hoarse voice due to lung dryness and yin vacuity. To be effective for these conditions, however, it must be taken regularly over a period of time.

Apricot Kernel & Pear Tea (*Xing Li Yin Cha*)

Apricot kernel, *i.e.*, Semen Pruni Armeniacae (*Xing Ren*)	10 grams
Large pear, *i.e.*, Fructus Pyrus Communis (*Da Li*)	1 fruit
Crystal sugar (*Bing Tang*)	Amount to taste

Method of administration: Remove the peel and tip from the apricot kernels and then pound into pieces. Core the pear and chop into cubes. Place the apricot kernels and pear into a pot, add water, and boil. When cooked, add the crystal sugar and allow to dissolve. Use 1 packet per day. Drink this freely as a tea at any time.

Functions: Moistens the lungs and stops cough

Indications: This tea is suitable for the treatment of dry heat acute tracheitis and cough.

Bronchial Asthma Teas

Bronchial asthma is a commonly encountered respiratory condition. Causative factors may include hypersensitivity to an environmental or seasonal allergen, infection, cold, fatigue, or emotional stress. In TCM, bronchial asthma is categorized as "wheezing and dyspnea" and is generally divided into vacuity and repletion patterns. Its main clinical symptoms are wheezing, dyspnea, and cough with sticky-natured phlegm. During attacks, the individual may sit up straight in an effort to breath. This may be accompanied by a cold sweat on the forehead. The lips may be purplish blue and the facial expression is pained. Such attacks may last hours or even days. In treating bronchial or allergic asthma, it is important to coordinate the proper herbal tea with the patient's

TCM pattern. In Chinese medicine, different treatments are also given during acute attacks and during remissions in order to prevent further attacks.

Calm Dyspnea Tea (*Ping Chuan Cha*)

Herba Ephedrae (*Ma Huang*)	3 grams
Cortex Phellodendri (*Huang Bai*)	4.5 grams
Semen Ginkgonis Bilobae (*Yin Guo*)	15 nuts
Tea leaves, *i.e.*, Folium Camelliae Theae (*Cha Ye*)	6 grams
White sugar (*Bai Tang*)	30 grams

Method of administration: Pound the ginkgo nuts into pieces. Place the first four ingredients in a pot and boil with water. Discard the dregs, save the liquid, and add white sugar. Use 1 packet 2 times per day. Drink this tea during attacks and when breathing is difficult.

Functions: Diffuses the lungs and depuratively downbears, calms dyspnea and stops cough

Indications: This tea is suitable for acute episodes of wheezing and dyspnea, *i.e.*, allergic, bronchial dyspnea.

Hawthorn & Walnut Tea (*Zha Tao Cha*)

Hawthorn fruit, *i.e.*, Fructus Crataegi (*Shan Zha*)	50 grams
Walnut, *i.e.*, Semen Juglandis Regiae (*Hu Tao Ren*)	150 grams
White sugar (*Bai Tang*)	200 grams

Method of administration: Soak the walnuts for half an hour, rinse well, and add water. Use a stone grinder to grind this mixture into a thick liquid. Place this liquid in a container, add water to dilute it, and stir evenly. Wash the hawthorn fruit well. The fruit should be patted to pieces. Place in a pot, add water, and boil over a medium fire 3 times, each time for 20 minutes. Discard the dregs and save the liquid. The remaining liquid should total a concentrate of 1,000ml. Wash the pot well, place the pot on the fire, add the hawthorn fruit juice and the white sugar, and then stir. When the sugar has melted, slowly add the thick walnut liquid, stirring continually while pouring. Cook this mixture until it starts to boil slightly. Then pour into a bowl. This tea should be taken often.

Functions: Supplements the lungs and kidneys and engenders liquid

Indications: This tea is suitable for lung vacuity cough and dyspnea, asthma, kidney vacuity impotence, low back pain, depletion of liquids, oral thirst, dry stool, food accumulation, reduced food intake, blood stasis scanty menstruation, and abdominal pain. It should be taken in between acute attacks.

Tangerine Peel Tea (*Chen Pi Cha*)

Tangerine peel, *i.e.,* Pericarpium Citri Reticulatae (*Ju Pi*)	Amount to taste
White sugar (*Bai Tang*)	Amount to taste

Note: It is best to use fresh, not aged tangerine peel.

Method of administration: Wash the tangerine peel well and tear into small pieces. Place in a cup, pour boiling water over it, and soak well. Discard the dregs, retain the liquid, add sugar to taste, and stir evenly.

Functions: Normalizes qi and stops cough, transforms phlegm and fortifies the stomach, disperses summerheat and eliminates pestilence

Indications: This tea is suitable for spleen vacuity/stomach weakness and cough and asthma. It can also beautify the skin.

Ginseng & Walnut Tea (*Ren Shen Hu Tao Cha*)

Ginseng, *i.e.,* Radix Panacis Ginseng (*Ren Shen*)	4 grams
Walnut, *i.e.,* Semen Juglandis Regiae (*Hu Tao Rou*)	4 pieces

Method of administration: Pound the ginseng and walnut into pieces, place them in a pot, and boil with water over a slow fire. This should make 400ml of concentrated liquid. Drink 1 packet per day, taken at any time. The ginseng and walnut can also be chewed and eaten.

Functions: Fortifies the spleen and supplements the kidneys, absorbs the qi and calms dyspnea

Indications: This tea is suitable for chronic dyspnea due to spleen/kidney vacuity. This typically varies in its severity from light to serious. It is accompanied by a yellow, somber, lusterless facial complexion, more breathing out, less breathing in, breathing with an open mouth and by lifting the shoulders, a pale tongue, and a deep, fine, forceless pulse. This tea should be taken between acute attacks.

2
Gastrointestinal Diseases

Stomachache Teas

Stomachache is also called epigastric pain and is commonly seen in acute and chronic gastritis, gastric ulcer or duodenal ulcer, as well as in neurosis. The dominant symptom is frequent pain occurring in the epigastric area. It is usually due to emotional depression, unsmooth liver qi, uncontrolled diet, and stomach vacuity with contraction of cold. If the liver qi invades the stomach, distention and pain occur in the epigastrium and there are attacks of pain that link with the lateral coastal region. Belching and sour vomiting are usually due to emotional changes. If the spleen and stomach are vacuous and cold, dull pain occurs in the epigastrium, clear water is vomited, the patient favors warmth and fears cold. This type of pain decreases with pressure and the obtainment of warmth. Accumulation and stagnation of food is usually due to excessive eating and drinking or unclean food and drink. Its symptoms are oppression, distention, and pain in the epigastrium, belching, scanty food intake, nausea, vomiting, possible borborygmus, and/or diarrhea. The following tea formulas should be prescribed based on TCM pattern discrimination and the signs and symptoms of the individual condition, not on the basis of stomach pain alone.

Old Ginger Tea (*Lao Jiang Cha*)

Uncooked ginger, *i.e.*, Rhizoma Zingiberis (*Sheng Jiang*)	250 grams
Brown sugar (*Hong Tang*)	250 grams

Note: Old here means that this formula is ancient, not that the ginger is old.

Method of administration: Pound the juice out of the fresh ginger and discard the dregs. Steam this juice in a double boiler, add the brown sugar, and allow it to dissolve. Make a paste or cream to be used for 8 doses. Each day, take 1 dose each in the morning and evening, dissolved in a cup of hot water.

Functions: Warms the middle and scatters cold

Indications: This tea is suitable for cold accumulation in the stomach. This pain in the epigastrium is due to insufficient stomach yin, internal damage due to cold drinks, and yin cold depression and binding. The pain is worse upon encountering cold. The other signs and symptoms are counterflow chilling of the hands and feet, clear, uninhibited stool and urination, and excessive saliva.

Fortify the Stomach Tea (*Jian Wei Cha*)

Radix Cynanchi Paniculati (*Xu Chang Qing*)	4.5 grams
Radix Glehniae Littoralis (*Bei Sha Shen*)	3 grams
Red tangerine peel, *i.e.*, Exocarpium Citri Erythrocarpae (*Ju Hong*)	3 grams
Peony root, *i.e.*, Radix Albus Paeoniae Lactiflorae (*Bai Shao*)	3 grams
Uncooked licorice root, *i.e.*, uncooked Radix Glycyrrhizae Uralensis (*Sheng Gan Cao*)	2 grams
Rose flower, *i.e.*, Flos Rosae Rugosae (*Mei Gui Hua*)	1.5 grams
Black Tea, *i.e.*, prepared Folium Camelliae Theae (*Hong Cha*)	1.5 grams

Method of administration: Grind the above ingredients into a coarse powder. Then soak them in boiling water. Take 1 packet per day with 3 months equaling 1 course of treatment.

Functions: Fortifies the spleen and warms the middle, courses the liver and quickens the blood

Indications: This tea is suitable for the treatment of vacuity cold gastritis with dull pain in the epigastrium which is aggravated by cold and relieved by warmth and pressure.

Ulcer Tea (*Kui Yang Cha*)

Tea leaves, *i.e.*, Folium Camelliae Theae (*Cha Ye*)	250 grams
White sugar (*Bai Tang*)	250 grams

Method of administration: Place the above two ingredients into a pot, add water, and boil twice. After it cools and settles, discard the dregs and store the liquid in a clean, covered container in a dry place. After 6-12 days, if the color looks like old wine and the congealed surface looks like a net, the liquid can be taken. If the surface has not congealed, allow 2 additional days. Heat the tea and take twice daily, 1 spoonful in the morning and 1 spoonful in the evening.

Functions: Harmonizes the middle and transforms dampness, disperses inflammation and closes the mouth of ulcerous sores

Indications: This tea is suitable for gastric ulcer and duodenal ulcer.

Note: This obviously describes a fermentation of tea with the netlike material floating on the surface being a fungal growth. This is the same as the very popular *Kombucha* "mushrooms" which have gained so much space in the popular press in the last couple of years. In China, rather than being the universal panacea many Westerners take it for, this tea is specifically used for the treatment of gastric and duodenal ulcers.

Licorice & Tangerine Tea (*Gan Ju Cha*)

Tangerine peel, *i.e.*, Pericarpium Citri Reticulatae (*Ju Pi*)	10 grams
Licorice root, *i.e.*, Radix Glycyrrhizae Uralensis (*Gan Cao*)	5 grams

Method of administration: Rinse these two ingredients well and tear the tangerine peels into pieces. Place these ingredients into a cup and soak in boiled water. Use 1 packet per day taken at any time.

Functions: Fortifies the spleen and rectifies the qi

Indications: This tea is suitable for the treatment of peptic ulcers with vomiting and excessive gastric secretion due to spleen vacuity weakness.

Honey & Safflower Tea (*Feng Mi Hong Cha*)

Safflower, *i.e.*, Flos Carthami Tinctorii (*Hong Hua*)	5 grams
Honey (*Feng Mi*)	Amount to taste
Brown sugar (*Hong Tang*)	Amount to taste

Method of administration: Place the 5 grams of safflowers in a thermos and then add boiling water. Cover and let the herb soak for 10 minutes. Add the honey and brown sugar. Use 1 packet per day. Drink while still hot or warm.

Functions: Harmonizes the stomach and disinhibits the intestines, stops pain and gets rid of open sores

Indications: This tea is suitable for gastric and duodenal ulcers as evidenced by the TCM pattern of blood stasis. This includes localized or fixed, sharp, intense pain, black, tarry stools, static spots or macules on the tongue or a purplish tongue, and a wiry, choppy pulse.

Eclipta & Red Date Tea (*Han Lian Hong Zao Cha*)

Fresh Herba Ecliptae Prostratae (*Xian Han Lian Cao*)	50 grams
Red Dates, *i.e.*, Fructus Ziziphi Jujubae (*Hong Zao*)	8 to 10 pieces

Method of administration: Boil the above two herbs in 2 bowls of water down to 1 bowlful. Discard the dregs and save the liquid. Take 1 packet per day in 2 divided doses.

Functions: Supplements the liver and kidneys and nourishes yin, supplements the blood and stops bleeding

Indications: This tea is suitable for bleeding due to gastric and duodenal ulcers and hemorrhagic anemia. In this case, the bleeding is due to blood heat in turn due to yin vacuity of the liver and kidneys. The signs and symptoms of this pattern are flushed red cheeks, especially in the late afternoon and early evening, night sweats, tinnitus, dizziness, low back and knee pain and weakness, a red tongue with scanty coating, and a fine, wiry, rapid pulse which is especially fine in the left bar and cubit positions. This formula has a good therapeutic effect.

Rose & Finger Citron Tea (*Mei Gui Fo Shou Cha*)

Rose flower, *i.e.*, Flos Rosae Rugosae (*Mei Gui Hua*)   6 grams
Finger citron fruit, *i.e.*, Fructus Citri Sacrodactylis (*Fo Shou*)   10 grams

Method of administration: Place the above two ingredients in a cup and soak in boiled water for 5 minutes. Take warm, 1 packet per day at any time.

Functions: Rectifies the qi and resolves depression, harmonizes the stomach and relieves pain

Indications: This tea is suitable for liver/stomach disharmony with lateral costal pain and distention, pain in the epigastrium, belching, and reduced food intake. The pain is worse under emotional stress and there is a darkish tongue with a wiry pulse.

Vomiting Teas

Vomiting is a common clinical symptom. Numerous diseases can cause impaired harmonious downbearing of the stomach and counterflow qi ascending upwards, and, in these cases, vomiting usually occurs. The clinical manifestations of cold vomiting are vomiting of clear drool, a desire for heat, absence of thirst, and coldness in the four limbs. The symptoms of hot vomiting are hot, foul or sour, bitter vomitus, a desire for cold drinks, thirst, and reddish yellow urination. The symptoms of liver qi invading the stomach are vomiting right after food intake, vomiting with chest oppression and pain in the coastal region. Vomiting due to a vacuous, weak spleen and stomach is characterized by difficult transformation of food and drink and frequent vomiting. Tea, because it has a bitter taste, descends and opens the stomach. Therefore, medicinal teas, *i.e.*, Tea leaves plus other medicinal herbs, are good for treating vomiting.

Fresh Ginger Harmonize the Stomach Tea (*Sheng Jiang He Wei Cha*)

Uncooked ginger, *i.e.*, uncooked Rhizoma Zingiberis (*Sheng Jiang*)   3 slices
Black Tea, *i.e.*, prepared Folium Camelliae Theae (*Hong Cha*)   1-3 grams

Method of administration: Chop the ginger into pieces or tiny threads. Place the ginger and black Tea in a cup and soak in boiling water for 3-5 minutes. Drink warm, 1-2 packets per day.

Functions: Warms the middle and harmonizes the stomach, downbears counterflow and stops vomiting

Indications: This tea is suitable for the treatment of vomiting and nausea.

Vinegar & Ginger Tea (*Cu Jiang Cha*)

Uncooked ginger, *i.e.*, uncooked Rhizoma Zingiberis (*Sheng Jiang*)   60 grams
Vinegar (*Cu*)   A suitable amount
Brown sugar (*Hong Tang*)   Amount to taste

Method of administration: Rinse the uncooked ginger and cut into slices. Soak these ginger slices in vinegar overnight. When the tea is to be taken, remove three slices of ginger each time and soak these with the brown sugar in boiling water for 5 minutes. Drink warm, 2 packets per day.

Functions: Warms the middle and harmonizes the stomach, downbears counterflow and stops vomiting

Indications: This tea is suitable for treatment of loss of appetite, stomach reflux, and pain in the epigastrium due to stomach cold.

Radish Leaf Tea (*Luo Bo Ye Cha*)

White radish leaf, *i.e.*, Folium Raphani Sativi (*Luo Bo Ye*)   100 grams

Method of administration: Pound these leaves to pieces or smash them into a pulp. Place in a cup, pour in boiling water, and drink.

Functions: Disperses food and transforms stagnation, fortifies the spleen and harmonizes the stomach

Indications: This tea is suitable for treating nausea and vomiting as well as internal damage due to the seven affects and externally contracted pathogenic qi that damages the spleen and stomach. This damage causes indigestion of accumulated food with symptoms of epigastric oppression and fullness, abdominal distention and pain, aversion to food, and vomiting right after food intake. Typically there is bad breath, a slimy tongue coating, and a slippery pulse.

Vinegar & Flour Tea (*Cu Mian Cha*)

Wheat flour (*Xiao Mai Mian*)   150 grams
Rice vinegar (*Mi Cu*)   A suitable amount
Tea leaves, *i.e.*, Folium Camelliae Theae (*Cha Ye*)   5 grams

Method of administration: Mix the wheat flour and vinegar to make bullet-sized balls. Boil or steam above water until they are cooked. When the balls are to be used, pour boiling water over the Tea leaves and eat the balls with the Tea water. Take twice per day, 1 ball each time. Continue to take the balls with the Tea water if the retching does not abate.

Functions: Harmonizes the stomach and downbears counterflow, relieves retching and stops vomiting

Indications: This tea is suitable for continuous vomiting.

Malted Barley & Hawthorn Fruit Tea (*Mai Ya Shan Zha Cha*)

Stir-fried malted barley, *i.e.*, Fructus Germinatus Hordei Vulgaris
    (*Chao Mai Ya*)   10 grams
Stir-fried hawthorn fruit slices, *i.e.*, stir-fried Fructus Crataegi
    (*Chao Shan Zha Pian*)   3 grams
Brown sugar (*Hong Tang*)   Amount to taste

Method of administration: Place the above three ingredients in a pot, add water, and boil. Discard the dregs and use the liquid. Use 1 packet per day. Drink it freely as a tea.

Functions: Disperses and abducts, stops vomiting

Indications: This tea is suitable for the treatment of food damage vomiting, epigastric and abdominal distention and fullness, belching of putrid gas and acid regurgitation, vomiting right after food intake, and vomiting of undigested, old food with sour and foul smell. Typically there is a slimy, white tongue coating and a slippery pulse.

Contraindications: Use malted barley with caution during pregnancy. It is contraindicated for nursing mothers since it dries up the milk.

Sugarcane & Ginger Juice Tea (*Gan Zhe Jiang Zhi Cha*)

Sugarcane (*Gan Zhe*)   1 section
Uncooked ginger, *i.e.*, uncooked Rhizoma Zingiberis (*Sheng Jiang*)   10 grams

Method of administration: Peel the sugarcane and squeeze out the juice. Extract the juice from the ginger and mix these two juices together stirring evenly. Use 1 packet per day. Drink as a tea at any time.

Functions: Downbears counterflow and stops vomiting

Indications: This tea is suitable for the treatment of stomach qi disharmony causing counterflow upward and vomiting, vexation and oppression within the chest, and frequent vomiting of phlegm drool.

Loquat & Phragmites Tea (*Pi Pa Lu Gen Cha*)

Loquat leaf, *i.e.*, Folium Eriobotryae Japonicae (*Pi Pa Ye*)   10-15 grams
Fresh Rhizoma Phragmitis Communis (*Xian Lu Gen*)   10 grams
White sugar (*Bai Tang*)   Amount to taste

Method of administration: Scrub the loquat leaves clean of any "hairs" or fur and then toast until dry. Place it and the phragmites in a pot and then boil with water. Discard the dregs and save the liquid. A small amount of white sugar can be added if desired. An alternate method is to place these ingredients in a cup and pour boiling water over them. This may be taken warm as a tea.

Functions: Clears heat and harmonizes the stomach

Indications: This tea is suitable for stomach heat with loss of harmonious downbearing. Instead, the qi counterflows upward and causes vomiting.

Hiccough Teas

Hiccoughing is due to counterflow qi ascending and surging. Its main symptom is a repeated, short, frequent hiccoughing sound in the throat which the person is not able to consciously stop. Its cause is stomach qi counterflowing upward stirring the diaphragm. Occasional cases of hiccough are often due to drinking cold beverages or breathing in cold air. Hiccoughing may be stopped by stimulating a sneeze, holding the breath, breathing into a paper bag, or diverting one's attention. If the hiccoughs continue, the following medicinal teas are effective for checking them.

Persimmon Calyx Tea (*Shi Di Cha*)

Calyx Diospyros Khaki (*Shi Di*)	3 grams
Caulis Bambusae In Taeniis (*Zhu Ru*)	3 grams
Tea leaves, *i.e.*, Folium Camelliae Theae (*Cha Ye*)	10 grams

Method of administration: Soak the above three ingredients in hot, boiling water. Drink warm repeatedly.

Functions: Downbears counterflow and stops hiccough

Indications: This tea is suitable for stomach cold hiccough.

Bamboo Shavings & Phragmites Tea (*Zhu Ru Lu Gen Cha*)

Caulis Bambusae In Taeniis (*Zhu Ru*)	30 grams
Rhizoma Phragmitis Communis (*Lu Gen*)	30 grams
Uncooked ginger, *i.e.*, uncooked Rhizoma Zingiberis (*Sheng Jiang*)	3 slices

Method of administration: Boil the above three ingredients. Discard the dregs and use the liquid. Use 1 packet per day. Drink this freely as a tea.

Functions: Clears heat, harmonizes the stomach, and downbears counterflow

Indications: This tea is suitable for stomach heat hiccough and hiccough after an illness.

Curing Hiccough Counterflow Medicinal Tea (*Zhi Er Ni Yao Cha*)

Hematitum (*Dai Zhe Shi*)	24 grams
Radix Auklandiae Lappae (*Mu Xiang*)	10 grams
Clove, *i.e.*, Flos Caryophylli (*Gong Ding Xiang*)	10 grams
Calyx Diospyros Khaki (*Shi Di*)	15 grams
Terra Flava Usta (*Fu Long Gan*)	150 grams

Method of administration: Boil the first four herbs together with water. Burn the last herb until red hot and then add to the boiling liquid. After the liquid settles, it may be drunk as a tea.

Functions: Downbears counterflow and stops hiccough

Indications: This tea is suitable for the treatment of hiccough in general.

Contraindications: Use with caution during pregnancy due to the strongly downbearing nature of Hematitum.

Hematemesis & Hemoptysis Teas

Blood ejection refers to spitting up blood from the mouth. It covers both the hacking of blood from the respiratory tract and the retching of blood from the digestive tract. There are a variety of causes for blood ejection in Chinese medicine. One is exuberant anger. This causes qi counterflow with liver fire seizing the stomach. Another cause is uncontrolled eating and drinking. This results in the stomach qi becoming damaged and deficient. A third cause is impact injury. This can break the vessels and network vessels. A fourth cause is overuse or wrongful use of cool and cold medicines. If these are taken to excess, they may produce vacuity cold internally. All these types of bleeding are due to blood not returning to the channels with counterflow of the stomach thus ejecting it outward. This is why it is called blood ejection. In addition, individuals with profuse hematemesis usually have black, tarry stools or melena.

Imperata & Ophiopogon Tea (*Mao Gen Mai Men Dong Cha*)

Rhizoma Imperatae Cylindricae (*Bai Mao Gen*)	30 grams
Tuber Ophiopogonis Japonici (*Mai Men Dong*)	30 grams
Crystal sugar (*Bing Tang*)	Amount to taste

Method of administration: Rinse the above two herbs well and pound them thoroughly. Then boil with water, save the liquid, and add the crystal sugar. Use 1 packet per day. Drink freely as a tea.

Functions: Enriches yin and moistens dryness, cools the blood and stops bleeding

Indications: This tea is suitable for the treatment of lung dryness blood ejection and dry cough due to yin vacuity.

Lotus & Biota Beverage Tea (*Ou Bai Yin Cha*)

Uncooked Nodus Nelumbinis Nuciferae (*Sheng Ou Jie*)	500 grams
Cacumen Biotae Orientalis (*Ce Bai Ye*)	100 grams

Method of administration: Thoroughly pound the above two herbs and save the juice. Add warm water to the juice and drink it as a tea.

Functions: Cools the blood and stops bleeding

Indications: This tea is suitable for the treatment of hematemesis, epistaxis, hemoptysis, and hematuria.

Lotus Flower Tea (*Lian Hua Cha*)

Lotus flower, *i.e.*, Flos Nelumbinis Nuciferae (*Lian Hua*)	6 grams
Green Tea, *i.e.*, Folium Camelliae Theae (*Lu Cha*)	3 grams

Method of administration: Dry the flowers in a cool place and then grind them and the green Tea into a fine powder. This powder may be made into tea bags or soak the powder in a cup. Use 1 packet per day soaked in boiling water for 5 minutes.

Functions: Clears summerheat and quiets the heart, cools the blood and stops bleeding

Indications: This tea is suitable for the treatment of summerheat vexation of the heart, hemoptysis, hematemesis, excessive menstruation, and abdominal pain due to static blood.

Two Fresh (Ingredients) Tea (*Er Xian Cha*)

Fresh Rhizoma Phragmitis Communis (*Xian Lu Gen*)   60 grams
Fresh Rhizoma Imperatae Cylindricae (*Xian Mao Gen*)   30 grams

Method of administration: Rinse the above two herbs well and then dry them in a cool place. Then chop into pieces and place in a pot. Bring to a boil several times. Discard the dregs and drink the liquid as a tea.

Functions: Clears heat, cools the blood, and stops bleeding

Indications: This tea is suitable for the treatment of epistaxis, spontaneous external bleeding, blood in the urine, blood in the stool, lung heat dyspnea and fullness, thirst, fever, and chest pain.

Abdominal Pain Teas

In TCM, abdominal pain typically occurs in relationship to diarrhea, intestinal abscess, parasitic disease, and various gynecological diseases. It is usually caused by contraction of cold evils or collection and stagnation of food and drink. Clinically, it is divided into two types—vacuity and repletion. In repletion patterns of abdominal pain, the abdomen refuses pressure or the pain is worse after food intake. In addition, there is abdominal distention, constipation, nausea, and vomiting. In vacuity patterns, the abdominal pain likes pressure or the pain is less after food intake. Further, there is no distention and the abdomen feels better when heat is applied to it. The following medicinal tea formulas should be chosen based on TCM pattern discrimination depending on the signs and symptoms of the individual person.

Hyacinth Bean Tea (*Bian Dou Cha*)

Hyacinth bean, *i.e.*, Semen Dolichoris Lablab (*Bian Dou*)   30 pieces

Method of administration: Pound the hyacinth beans into a liquid. Place in a pot, add water, and boil. Drink frequently as a tea.

Functions: Moves the qi and transforms dampness, clears heat and drains fire

Indications: This tea is suitable for damp heat abdominal pain due to damp heat brewing and binding in the spleen and stomach. The abdominal pain is periodic, meaning it comes and goes, it refuses pressure, and retching and vomiting occur periodically along with other symptoms, such as constipation or dysentery.

Leechee Nut Tea (*Li Zhi He Cha*)

Leechee nut, *i.e.*, Semen Litchi Chinensis (*Li Zhi He*)   15 grams
Tangerine seed, *i.e.*, Semen Citri Reticulatae (*Ju He*)   10 grams
Brown sugar (*Hong Tang*)   Amount to taste

Method of administration: Boil the above two herbs and save the liquid. Add brown sugar to the liquid and allow it to dissolve. Drink this freely as a tea.

Functions: Moves the qi and scatters cold

Indications: This tea is suitable for the treatment of cold-feeling abdominal pain. This pain is continuous. It likes warmth and it likes pressure. The facial complexion is yellowish white and there is no thirst in the mouth. In this case, cold stagnation blocks the free flow of qi, thus resulting in pain.

Two Pits Tea (*Er Ren Cha*)

Peach kernel, *i.e.*, Semen Pruni Persicae (*Tao Ren*)	9 grams
Prune kernel, *i.e.*, Semen Pruni (*Yu Li Ren*)	6 grams
Tails of Radix Angelicae Sinensis (*Dang Gui Wei*)	5 grams
Fennel seed, *i.e.*, Fructus Foeniculi Vulgaris (*Xiao Hui Xiang*)	1 gram
Saffron, *i.e.*, Stigma Croci Sativi (*Zang Hong Hua*)	1.5 grams

Method of administration: Place the above herbs in a pot and bring to a boil several times with water. Drink the resulting tea slowly at any time of the day.

Functions: Quickens the blood and moves the qi

Indications: This tea is suitable for the treatment of qi stagnation and blood stasis obstructing the vessels and hindering free flow. This results in obstruction of the large intestine which then causes distention and fullness with inhibited defecation and urination.

Harmonize the Spleen Tea (*He Pi Cha*)

Powdered Sclerotium Poriae Cocos (*Fu Ling Fen*)	10 grams
Peony root, *i.e.*, Radix Albus Paeoniae Lactiflorae (*Bai Shao*)	10 grams
Earth stir-fried Rhizoma Atractylodis Macrocephalae (*Tu Chao Bai Zhu*)	6 grams
Mixed-fried Licorice root, *i.e.*, mix-fried Radix Glycyrrhizae Uralensis (*Zhi Gan Cao*)	3 grams

Method of administration: Boil the above four ingredients in water. Discard the dregs and drink the liquid. Use 1 packet per day.

Functions: Fortifies the spleen and nourishes the stomach, relaxes tension and stops pain

Indications: This tea is suitable for the treatment of spleen and stomach vacuity with poor appetite, loose stools, and aching and pain within the abdomen.

Diarrhea Teas

In TCM, diarrhea is also called abdominal diarrhea. Its main symptom is increased frequency of defecation with loose stools. It is usually caused by the prevalence of damp evils and disharmony of the spleen and stomach. The causes are differentiated as damp heat, cold damp contraction, spleen/stomach vacuity, or kidney yang insufficiency. Thus, in TCM, diarrhea is differentiated into the patterns of damp heat pouring downward, cold and dampness damaging the spleen, spleen vacuity diarrhea, or life-gate fire decline. This latter pattern is also sometimes referred to as cock-crow or fifth watch diarrhea, *i.e.*, diarrhea before dawn. In Western medicine, diarrhea may be due to acute or chronic enteritis, intestinal tuberculosis, gastrointestinal neural dysfunction, infections, a reaction to various medications, psychogenic factors, and colitis. Diagnosis and treatment in TCM are given based on the overall analysis of the patient's pattern and their signs and symptoms.

Stop Diarrhea Tea (*Zhi Xie Cha*)

Green Tea, *i.e.*, Folium Camelliae Theae (*Lu Cha*)	9 grams
Honeysuckle flower, *i.e.*, Flos Lonicerae Japonicae (*Jin Yin Hua*)	9 grams
Rose flower, *i.e.*, Flos Rosae Rugosae (*Mei Gui Hua*)	6 grams
Tangerine peel, *i.e.*, Pericarpium Citri Reticulatae (*Chen Pi*)	6 grams
Jasmine flower, *i.e.*, Flos Jasmini (*Mo Li Hua*)	3 grams
Licorice root, *i.e.*, Radix Glycyrrhizae Uralensis (*Gan Cao*)	3 grams

Method of administration: Soak the above herbs in boiling water and cover tightly with a lid for 10-12 minutes. Use 1 packet per day. Drink this tea 3-5 times per day. Children should take a reduced amount.

Functions: Disperses inflammation and combats bacteria, promotes contraction and secures the intestines, rectifies the qi and relieves pain, disperses and transforms food accumulation (especially meat), quickens the blood and stops bleeding, strengthens the heart and disinhibits the urine, clears heat and resolves toxins

Indications: This tea is suitable for the treatment of acute or chronic enteritis, bacillary dysentery, and diarrhea exhibiting a damp heat pattern with qi stagnation and a possible element of food stagnation.

Two Flowers Tea (*Er Hua Cha*)

Black Tea, *i.e.*, prepared Folium Camelliae Theae (*Hong Cha*)	10 grams
Honeysuckle flower, *i.e.,* Flos Lonicerae Japonicae (*Jin Yin Hua*)	10 grams
Rose flower, *i.e.*, Flos Rosae Rugosae (*Mei Gui Hua*)	6 grams
Licorice root, *i.e.*, Radix Glycyrrhizae Uralensis (*Gan Cao*)	6 grams
Rhizoma Coptidis Chinensis (*Huang Lian*)	6 grams

Method of administration: Boil the above herbs and reserve the liquid. Drink it immediately after preparing.

Functions: Clears heat and resolves toxins, moves the qi and relieves pain, secures the intestines and stops diarrhea

Indications: This tea is suitable for the treatment of acute or chronic enteritis, dysentery, and diarrhea due to damp heat. Its ability to clear heat is stronger than the preceding tea.

Pomegranate Leaf Tea (*Shi Liu Ye Cha*)

Pomegranate leaf, *i.e.*, Folium Punicae Granati (*Shi Liu Ye*)	60 grams
Uncooked ginger, *i.e.*, uncooked Rhizoma Zingiberis (*Sheng Jiang*)	15 grams
Salt (*Yan*)	30 grams

Method of administration: Stir-fry the three ingredients until they are black and then boil them in water. Take 1 packet per day, drinking the tea while it is warm, 1 dose in the morning and 1 dose in the afternoon.

Functions: Warms the middle and stops diarrhea

Indications: This tea is suitable for the treatment of acute gastroenteritis of the cold diarrhea pattern type.

Plantain Seed Tea (*Che Qian Zi Cha*)

Stir-fried plantain seeds, *i.e.*, stir-fried Semen Plantaginis (*Chao Che Qian Zi*)	10 grams
Black Tea, *i.e.*, prepared Folium Camelliae Theae (*Hong Cha*)	3 grams

Method of administration: Soak these two ingredients in boiling water and cover for 10 minutes. To make a stronger tea, another method is to boil the two ingredients in water. Take 1-2 packets per day. Drink this tea warm 2 times each day.

Functions: Fortifies the spleen and disinhibits water, transforms dampness and stops diarrhea

Indications: This tea is suitable for the treatment of spleen vacuity water diarrhea. This formula is mainly for disinhibiting urination, *i.e.*, promoting urination, and solidifying the stools in order to stop diarrhea.

Polished Rice & Ginger Tea (*Jing Mi Jiang Cha*)

Tea leaves, *i.e.*, Folium Camelliae Theae (*Cha Ye*)	15 grams
Uncooked ginger, *i.e.*, uncooked Rhizoma Zingiberis (*Sheng Jiang*)	3 grams
Polished rice, *i.e.*, Semen Oryzae Sativae (*Jing Mi*)	30 grams

Method of administration: Rinse the rice well, add uncooked ginger, and boil in Tea water. Drink warm, 1 packet per day.

Functions: Clears heat and resolves toxins, fortifies the spleen and disinhibits urination

Indications: This tea is suitable for the treatment of chronic enteritis and enduring, incessant diarrhea. It is especially effective for spleen/stomach vacuity and coldness caused by constant diarrhea.

Umeboshi Sweet Tea (*Wu Mei Tian Cha*)

Umeboshi, *i.e.*, Fructus Pruni Mume (*Wu Mei*)	5 grams
Radix Ledebouriellae Divaricatae (*Fang Feng*)	8 grams
Radix Angelicae Sinensis (*Dang Gui*)	8 grams
White sugar (*Bai Tang*)	Amount to taste

Note: Umeboshi refers to a fermented Asian plum. In the West, this is sold most commonly under its Japanese name: umeboshi.

Method of administration: Wash the umeboshi plum well, place it with the other ingredients in a cup, and soak in boiling water. Use 1 packet per day. This may be drunk at any time of the day.

Functions: Promotes contraction and engenders liquid

Indications: This tea is suitable for the treatment of diarrhea caused by allergic enteritis or, in other words, diarrhea due to food allergies.

Dysentery Teas

Dysentery is a common acute intestinal tract disorder that often occurs in China during the late summer and autumn. However, Westerners traveling in underdeveloped and especially tropical countries may catch this disease at any time of the year. Its main symptoms are abdominal pain, cramping and rectal tenesmus, red and white purulent blood, *i.e.*, mucous and blood in the stools, with 10 or more bowel movements per day. The difference between diarrhea and dysentery is that dysentery is characterized by inflammation of the mucous membranes and is due to bacterial, viral, parasitic, protozoan, or chemical causes. Diarrhea refers only to frequent watery bowel movements and may or may not involve inflammation. The number of times of defecation are usually fewer per day than with dysentery. In TCM, dysentery is usually caused by externally contracted damp heat, epidemic toxic qi, and internal damage due to drinking and eating of raw, cold foods. These then collect and become stagnant in the intestines. Thus conveyance and conduction lose their normalcy resulting in this condition. The Chinese disease category of dysentery includes Western medicine's diseases of acute and chronic bacillary dysentery and amoebic dysentery.

Kill Germs & Stop Dysentery Tea (*Sha Jun Zhi Li Cha*)

Green Tea, *i.e.*, Folium Camelliae Theae (*Lu Cha*)   2 grams

Method of administration: Boil the green Tea in 100ml of water until 40-50ml of liquid is left. Drink immediately after decoction, 4 times per day.

Functions: Disperses inflammation and kills germs, stops dysentery

Indications: This tea is suitable for the treatment of bacillary dysentery and enteritis.

Treating Dysentery Rapidly & Effectively Tea (*Zhi Li Su Xiao Cha*)

Fine Tea, *i.e.*, Folium Camelliae Theae (*Xi Cha*)   9 grams
Betel nut, *i.e.*, Semen Arecae Catechu (*Bing Lang*)   9 grams
Salt (*Yan*)   A suitable amount

Method of administration: Briefly stir-fry the Tea leaves and salt and then discard the salt. Boil the Tea and betel nut in water. Drink warm. Use 1-2 packets per day.

Functions: Removes congestion and stagnation, eliminates damp heat, and stops dysentery

Indications: This tea is suitable for the treatment of all the symptoms of dysentery but especially for relieving tenesmus.

Purslane & White Sugar Tea (*Ma Chi Xian Bai Tang Cha*)

Purslane, *i.e.*, Herba Portulacae Oleraceae (*Ma Chi Xian*)	50 grams
White sugar (*Bai Tang*)	30 grams
Tea leaves, *i.e.*, Folium Camelliae Theae (*Cha Ye*)	10 grams

Method of administration: Place the above three ingredients together in a pot. Briefly boil them in water. Use 1 packet per day. This tea should be drunk continuously for 3-5 days.

Functions: Clears heat and disinhibits urination, resolves toxins and stops dysentery

Indications: This tea is suitable for the treatment of damp heat pattern bacillary dysentery.

Hawthorn Stop Dysentery Tea (*Shan Zha Zhi Li Cha*)

Hawthorn fruit (partially cooked), *i.e.*, Fructus Crataegi (*Shan Zha*)	60 grams
Tea leaves, *i.e.*, Folium Camelliae Theae (*Cha Ye*)	15 grams
Uncooked ginger, *i.e.*, uncooked Rhizoma Zingiberis (*Sheng Jiang*)	6 grams
Brown sugar (*Hong Tang*)	15 grams
White sugar (*Bai Tang*)	15 grams

Method of administration: Boil the hawthorn fruit, Tea leaves, and ginger in water for 10-15 minutes. Discard the dregs and save the liquid. Add the brown and white sugar to the liquid. Drink 2 packets per day at any time.

Functions: Clears heat and disperses stagnation, transforms dampness and disperses inflammation, stops dysentery

Indications: This tea is suitable for damp heat dysentery, bacillary dysentery, and enteritis.

Contraindications: Melons, gourds, fruit, fish, *i.e.*, seafood, greasy, glutinous, and hard foods are forbidden while taking this tea. Actually, they are forbidden with this pattern and disease.

Two Aged (Ingredients) Stop Dysentery Tea (*Er Chen Zhi Li Cha*)

Old Tea leaves, *i.e.*, aged Folium Camelliae Theae (*Chen Cha Ye*) 10 grams
Tangerine peel, *i.e.*, Pericarpium Citri Reticulatae (*Chen Pi*) 10 grams
Uncooked ginger, *i.e.*, uncooked Rhizoma Zingiberis (*Sheng Jiang*) 7 grams

Method of administration: Boil the above three ingredients in water for 5-10 minutes. Drink the liquid warm. Use 2-3 packets per day, drunk at any time.

Functions: Clears heat and disinhibits dampness, harmonizes the middle and rectifies the qi, stops dysentery

Indications: This tea is suitable for heat dysentery, cramping, and tenesmus with pus and blood. This formula is especially effective for this type of dysentery.

Agrimony Tea (*Xian He Cha*)

Herba Agimoniae Pilosae (*Xian He Cao*) 10 grams
Old Tea leaves, *i.e.*, aged Folium Camelliae Theae (*Chen Cha Ye*) 10 grams

Method of administration: Rinse the above two ingredients, boil in water, and then use the liquid. Drink warm, 1 packet per day at any time.

Functions: Clears heat and disinhibits dampness, stops dysentery and stops bleeding

Indications: This tea is suitable for the treatment of red and white dysentery. This means dysentery with pus and blood in the stools.

Umeboshi Stop Dysentery Tea (*Wu Mei Zhi Li Cha*)

Umeboshi (without pit), *i.e.*, Fructus Pruni Mume (*Wu Mei*)   1 piece
Tea leaves, *i.e.*, Folium Camelliae Theae (*Cha Ye*)   A suitable amount

Method of administration: Burn or mix-fry the umeboshi plum into a powder and store for later use. When needed, boil 6 grams of this powder along with the Tea leaves in water. Take 2-3 times per day.

Functions: Constrains and astringes, stops dysentery and stanches bleeding

Indications: This tea is suitable for the treatment of dysentery with pus and blood.

Porridge Tea (*Zhou Cha*)

Tea leaves, *i.e.*, Folium Camelliae Theae (*Cha Ye*)   10 grams
Polished rice, *i.e.*, Semen Oryzae Sativae (*Jing Mi*)   50 grams
White sugar (*Bai Tang*)   Amount to taste

Method of administration: Boil the Tea with water into a strong liquid of about 1,000ml. Add this liquid to the rice and season with white sugar. Then boil these three ingredients together with another 400ml of water until it becomes a pulpy, thick gruel. Use 1 packet per day. Drink warm in 2 doses per day.

Functions: Fortifies the spleen and disinhibits dampness, boosts the qi and raises the spirit, stops dysentery

Indications: This tea is suitable for the treatment of acute and chronic dysentery and enteritis when associated with concomitant spleen vacuity.

Ginger & Umeboshi Tea (*Jiang Mei Cha*)

Uncooked ginger, *i.e.*, uncooked Rhizoma Zingiberis (*Sheng Jiang*)	10 grams
Umeboshi (without pit), *i.e.*, Fructus Pruni Mume (*Wu Mei*)	30 grams
Green Tea, *i.e.*, Folium Camelliae Theae (*Lu Cha*)	6 grams
Brown sugar (*Hong Tang*)	Amount to taste

Method of administration: Chop the ginger and umeboshi plum into thin threads. Then soak them and the green Tea in boiling water in a thermos. Cover tightly for half an hour. Then add the brown sugar. Drink warm. Use 1 packet taken in 3 divided doses per day.

Functions: Clears heat and engenders liquids, stops dysentery, disperses food, and warms the middle

Indications: This tea is suitable for the treatment of bacillary or amoebic dysentery when there is a combination of heat and cold, vacuity and repletion.

Red Date & Honey Tea (*Zao Mi Cha*)

Red dates, *i.e.*, Fructus Zizyphi Jujubae (*Hong Zao*)	10 pieces
Honey (*Feng Mi*)	50 grams
Green Tea, *i.e.*, Folium Camelliae Theae (*Lu Cha*)	10 grams

Method of administration: Chop and then boil the red dates for 15 minutes. Add the green Tea, boil briefly again, and strain the liquid. Add the honey to the liquid and stir till dissolved. Use 1 packet per day, taken once in the morning and once in the afternoon.

Functions: Clears heat and disinhibits dampness, kills germs and disperses inflammation, restrains and astringes and stops dysentery

Indications: This tea is suitable for the treatment of chronic bacillary dysentery accompanied by spleen vacuity.

Ancestral Poppy & Umeboshi Tea (*Zu Chuan Ying Mei Cha*)

Pericarpium Papaveris Somniferi (*Ying Su Ke*)	15 grams
Licorice root, *i.e.,* Radix Glycyrrhizae Uralensis (*Gan Cao*)	15 grams
Black Tea, *i.e.,* prepared Folium Camelliae Theae (*Hong Cha*)	15 grams
Brown sugar (*Hong Tang*)	15 grams
Umeboshi, *i.e.,* Fructus Pruni Mume (*Wu Mei*)	7 pieces
Black pepper, *i.e.,* Fructus Piperis Nigri (*Hu Jiao*)	7 pieces

Method of administration: Boil the above six ingredients in water twice. Put the liquid from the two boilings together and drink warm, 1 packet per day.

Functions: Astringes the intestines and stops dysentery

Indications: This tea is suitable for red and white dysentery and enduring dysentery. This is an ancestral tea handed down from generation to generation which has cured countless patients. However, it should only be used to treat cases of dysentery which have gone on for sometime without stopping due to kidney vacuity not astringing the intestines. If there is still exuberant heat and the intestines are astringed, this will only worsen the disease.

Hawthorn & Auklandia Tea (*Shan Zha Mu Xiang Cha*)

Black Tea, *i.e.,* prepared Folium Camelliae Theae (*Hong Cha*)	15 grams
Stir-fried hawthorn fruit, *i.e.,* stir-fried Fructus Crataegi (*Chao Shan Zha*)	25 grams
Radix Auklandiae Lappae (*Mu Xiang*)	6 grams
Sugar (*Tang*)	20 grams

Note: In red dysentery due to heat, use white sugar. In white dysentery due to spleen vacuity and dampness, use brown sugar. In red and white dysentery due to both heat and dampness, use half white and half brown sugar.

Method of administration: Boil the above ingredients in water until 500ml of liquid remain. Drink immediately, 1 packet in the morning and 1 packet in the evening.

Functions: Rectifies the qi and harmonizes the middle, disperses food and stops dysentery

Indications: This tea is suitable for bacillary dysentery due to food stagnation obstructing the free flow of the qi.

Habitual Constipation Teas

Habitual constipation refers to dry, hard stools and difficult defecation with infrequent evacuation. Often, 2-3 days go by without a bowel movement. In TCM, this illness is differentiated into righteous vacuity and evil repletion patterns. In qi vacuity with yang weakness constipation, there is no strength to push or evacuate the stools. In yin vacuity patterns with blood deficiency, there is intestinal dryness that causes constipation. In this case, there is not enough water to float the boat so to speak. Both of these vacuity patterns can be called yin binding. In repletion constipation, the causes may be heat, phlegm, and/or dampness congestion and binding or qi stagnation with no movement. These are called yang binding. During treatment, medicinal teas should be selected based on pattern discriminaton and the individual patient's signs and symptoms.

Senna Leaf Tea (*Fan Xie Ye Cha*)

Senna leaf, *i.e.*, Folium Sennae (*Fan Xie Ye*)   1-3 grams

Method of administration: Place this herb in a cup and soak in boiling water. Drink it frequently as a tea.

Functions: Drains heat, moves the stools, and abducts stagnation

Indications: This tea is suitable for the treatment of dry, bound stools, dry mouth, and a foul odor in the mouth, a red facial complexion, a hot body, short voidings of reddish urine, vexation and fullness, or pain in the abdomen.

Contraindications: Senna leaf is a purgative and has a strong laxative action that may be accompanied by abdominal pain. It is contraindicated during pregnancy, for nursing mothers, during menstruation, and in individuals who are weak. It is not suitable to use this formula long-term.

Cassia & Cistanches Tea (*Jue Ming Cong Rong Cha*)

Semen Cassiae Torae (*Jue Ming Zi*)	10 grams
Herba Cistanchis Deserticolae (*Rou Cong Rong*)	10 grams
Honey (*Feng Mi*)	Amount to taste

Method of administration: Stir-fry the cassia seeds and then grind into a fine powder. Soak the two herbs in boiling water and then filter them. Add honey to the resulting liquid and drink. Use 1 packet per day. Drink this freely as a tea.

Functions: Moistens the intestines and frees the stools

Indications: This tea is suitable for habitual constipation, constipation in the elderly, and constipation with dryness of the intestines.

Soybean Skin Tea (*Huang Dou Pi Cha*)

Soybean skins, *i.e.*, Cortex Seminis Sojae (*Huang Dou Pi*)	120 grams

Method of administration: Pulverize the soybeans and use the skin. Boil the skins in water and drink the resulting liquid after straining out the skins. Use 1 packet per day. Drink this freely as a tea.

Functions: Fortifies the spleen and loosens the middle, moistens dryness and frees the stools

Indicatons: This tea is suitable for the treatment of bound stool or habitual constipation due to spleen vacuity and fluid dryness.

Uncooked Rhubarb Tea (*Sheng Jun Cha*)

Uncooked rhubarb, *i.e.*, uncooked Radix Et Rhizoma Rhei (*Sheng Jun*)   4 grams
White sugar (*Bai Tang*)   Amount to taste

Method of administration: Soak the rhubarb in boiling water for 5 minutes. Then add the white sugar. Drink 1-2 packets per day at any time.

Functions: Clears heat and frees the flow of the bowels, drains downward and frees the stools

Indications: This tea is suitable for the treatment of stomach and intestine dryness and heat pattern constipation.

Contraindications: Rhubarb is a purgative and should be used with caution during pregnancy or postpartum. It is contraindicated in nursing mothers as its active ingredients can enter the milk and cause diarrhea in the baby.

Cassia Moisten the Intestines Tea (*Jue Ming Run Chang Cha*)

Semen Cassiae Torae (*Jue Ming Zi*)   30 grams

Method of administration: Stir-fry the cassia seeds to a proper degree. Then pulverize. Soak in boiling water for 5-10 minutes. Take 1 packet per day.

Functions: Moistens the intestines and frees the stools, lowers lipids and brightens the eyes

Indications: This tea is suitable for the treatment of constipation as well as hypertension and hyperlipemia due to liver repletion.

Sesame Oil & Honey Tea (*Xiang Mi Cha*)

Honey (*Feng Mi*)   65 grams
Roasted sesame oil (*Xiang You*)   35ml

Method of administration: Add the roasted sesame oil to the honey, pour in boiling water, and stir. Take once in the morning and once in the evening.

Functions: Moistens the intestines and frees the stools

Indications: This tea is suitable for the treatment of habitual constipation due to vacuity dryness.

Four Seed Free the Stools Tea (*Si Ren Tong Bian Cha*)

Stir-fried apricot seeds, *i.e.*, stir-fried Semen Pruni Armeniacae
   (*Chao Xing Ren*)   9 grams
Pinenuts, *i.e.*, Semen Pini (*Song Zi Ren*)   9 grams
Semen Cannabis Sativae (*Da Ma Ren*)   9 grams
Semen Biotae Orientalis (*Bai Zi Ren*)   9 grams

Method of administration: Grind the above four ingredients and place in a cup. Soak in boiling water and cover briefly. Use 1 packet per day. This tea may be drunk frequently.

Functions: Nourishes yin and moistens dryness, frees the stools

Indications: This tea is suitable for the treatment of yin vacuity and fluid dryness in the elderly.

Biota Seed & Honey Tea (*Bai Ren Mi Cha*)

Semen Biotae Orientalis (*Bai Zi Ren*)	15 grams
Honey (*Feng Mi*)	Amount to taste

Method of administration: Grind the biota seeds into pieces, boil with water, and drink the liquid. Add honey to the liquid to taste. Drink 1 packet per day.

Functions: Moistens the intestines and frees the stools, quiets the heart and sharpens the wits

Indications: This tea is suitable for the treatment of habitual constipation in the elderly or constipation accompanied with palpitations and insomnia due to yin vacuity and fluid dryness.

Prolapse of the Rectum Tea

Prolapse of the rectum refers to the downward falling of the rectum out of the anus. In TCM, this is usually due to enduring diarrhea, enduring dysentery, hemorrhoids, chronic cough, or overtaxation resulting in spleen vacuity and downward falling of central qi.

Ginger Slice Tea (*Jiang Pian Cha*)

Tea leaves, *i.e.*, Folium Camelliae Theae (*Cha Ye*)	1 handful
Uncooked ginger, *i.e.*, uncooked Rhizoma Zingiberis (*Sheng Jiang*)	7 slices

Method of administration: Boil the above two ingredients in water or soak in boiling water. Use 1-2 packets per day and drink while it is hot.

Functions: Warms the middle and disinhibits dampness, astringes the intestines and stops dysentery, secures desertion

Indications: This tea is suitable for prolapse of the rectum due to dysentery.

Hemorrhoid Teas

Hemorrhoids are a common problem. In China, there is a saying, "Nine out of ten people have hemorrhoids." Hemorrhoids are a type of varicosity. There are two types of hemorrhoid: internal and external. External hemorrhoids protrude beyond the boundary between the anus and the rectum and are not obvious until defecation is difficult. Then there is often pain. Internal hemorrhoids involve the veins inside the rectum line and do not protrude outside the anus. Their main symptom is bleeding upon defecation.

Artemisia Anomala Tea (*Liu Ji Nu Cha*)

Herba Artemisiae Anomalae (*Liu Ji Nu*)	No set amount
Tea leaves, *i.e.*, Folium Camelliae Theae (*Cha Ye*)	A suitable amount

Method of administration: Grind the artemisia anomala into a fine powder, place this powder in a container, and seal it for storage. Two to three times a day, use 3 grams of this powder, boiling it with water and the Tea leaves. Drink this tea while it is warm. Another method is to grind the first herb into a coarse powder and soak this powder and the Tea in boiling water for 15 minutes. The dosage and frequency are the same as in the first method.

Functions: Cools the blood and stops bleeding

Indications: This tea is suitable for blood in the stools or urine due to heat.

Day Lily Tea (*Jin Zhen Cai Cha*)

Day lily flowers, *i.e.*, Flos Hemerocallis (*Jin Zhen Cai*)	100 grams
Brown sugar (*Hong Tang*)	A suitable amount

Method of administration: Boil these two ingredients until the lily flowers are cooked. Then discard the dregs. Drink the resulting liquid in the morning when the stomach is empty. Take this tea continuously for several days.

Functions: Clears heat and disinhibits the urine, nourishes the blood and calms the liver

Indications: This tea is suitable for the treatment of hemorrhoid pain and bleeding due to heat in the blood, in turn due to liver depression. The symptoms of liver depression transforming heat are irritability, a bitter taste in the mouth, possible lateral costal pain, a red tongue with a thin, yellow coating, and a wiry, rapid pulse.

Wood Ear & Sesame Tea (*Mu Er Zhi Ma Cha*)

Black wood ear, *i.e.*, Exidia Auricula Judae (*Hei Mu Er*)   60 grams
Black sesame seeds, *i.e.*, black Semen Sesami Indici (*Hei Zhi Ma*)   15 grams
White sugar (*Bai Tang*)   Amount to taste

Method of administration: Place half of the black wood ears into a wok. Fry until they become black with a burnt smell. Then remove them from the wok. Stir-fry the sesame seeds until they smell fragrant. Add 1500ml of clear water and, at the same time, put in the cooked and uncooked wood ears. Boil for 30 minutes over a medium fire, remove the dregs, and filter with a double layer of gauze, pouring the liquid into a container for use. Each time, drink 100-120ml of this liquid with 20-25 grams of white granulated sugar (optional). Take 2-3 doses per day.

Functions: Cools the blood and stops bleeding, moistens the intestines and frees the stools

Indications: This tea is suitable for the treatment of blood heat hemafecia, hemorrhoidal bleeding, intestinal wind bleeding, and bloody dysentery.

3
Liver & Kidney Diseases

Drum Distention Teas

In TCM, drum distention refers to abdominal distention and swelling like a drum. This is accompanied by a pale, yellowish skin color. In the worst cases, the veins can be seen on the abdomen. This condition is usually caused by undisciplined eating and drinking, internal damage due to the seven emotions, infection by blood flukes, or as the result of some other disease. Western medicine's ascites due to cirrhosis of the liver or other diseases belongs to this disease category in TCM. This condition usually occurs in the advanced stage of other various diseases. If the disease condition is severe, the presenting pattern and its symptoms are complex and treatment is relatively difficult. The following medicinal teas should be used as adjunctive treatments only, nevertheless based on the patient's TCM pattern discrimination.

Plum Tea (*Li Zi Cha*)

Fresh plums (*Xian Li Zi*)	100-150 grams
Green Tea, *i.e.*, Folium Cameliae Theae (*Lu Cha*)	2 grams
Honey (*Feng Mi*)	25 grams

Method of administration: Open the plums and place in a pot. Add 320ml of water and boil for 3 minutes. Then add the Tea and honey. When the formula returns to a boil, turn off the heat, strain, and save the liquid. Use 1 packet per day. Take 1 dose in the morning and 1 dose in the evening.

Functions: Clears heat and disinhibits dampness, softens the liver and scatters nodulations

Indications: This tea is suitable for the treatment of cirrhosis with ascites.

Atractylodes & Immature Aurantium Tea (*Bai Zhu Zhi Shi Cha*)

Rhizoma Atractylodis Macrocephalae (*Bai Zhu*)	15 grams
Fructus Immaturus Aurantii (*Zhi Shi*)	45 grams

Method of administration: Boil the above two ingredients in water. Drink the tea made from 1 packet per day at any time.

Functions: Moves the qi and disperses swelling

Indications: This tea is suitable for the treatment of qi drum water swelling, *i.e.,* edema. It is better for ascites due to cirrhosis and late stage schistosomiasis drum distention associated with spleen vacuity and qi stagnation due to accumulated dampness.

Maple & Poplar Tea (*Feng Yang Cha*)

Maple leaves (*Feng Shu Ye*)	A suitable amount
Poplar leaves (*Yang Shu Ye*)	A suitable amount
Green Tea, *i.e.*, Folium Cameliae Theae (*Lu Cha*)	A suitable amount

Method of administration: Wash the fresh maple and poplar leaves well. Place them in hot water. Then, after a few minutes, remove them from the water. Dry the leaves in the sun for later use. Each day, use 1 handful (50-60 grams) of the maple and poplar leaves. Soaking them in boiling water for 15 minutes. The resulting tea may be taken at any time. Another method is to use fresh maple and poplar leaves (500 grams). Add 750ml water, boil for 10-15 minutes, and then add the green Tea (6 grams). Bring to a boil for 1 minute, discard the dregs, and use the liquid. Drink 100ml of this liquid 3 times per day for 20-30 days. This equals 1 course of treatment.

Functions: Disinhibits dampness and disperses swelling, kills worms and resolves toxins

Indications: This tea is suitable for the treatment of schistosomiasis, hepatosplenomegaly, and ascites.

Hepatitis Teas

Acute hepatitis accompanied by jaundice, *i.e.*, cholangiolitic hepatitis, belongs to the category of "jaundice" or "yellowing" in TCM. Its three main symptoms are a yellow skin color, yellow eyes, and yellow urine. This is usually due to the contraction of seasonal evils, uncontrolled diet, or damp heat. These then cause blockage within the middle burner which forces the bile to flow out of its normal course. It usually occurs suddenly, and, within a few days, the skin of the whole body is a bright yellow color. This is called yang jaundice. Yin jaundice is a transformation from yang jaundice if yang jaundice has lasted for a long time. Yin jaundice may also be due to devitalization of spleen yang, cold and dampness brewing internally, or ingestion of excessive cold food and drink. Its symptoms are dark or dim yellow color to the skin and eyes with fatigue and other symptoms of spleen vacuity and dampness.

Chronic hepatitis is a chronic inflammation of the liver. The course of the disease is generally from ½-1 year, although it can last for 10 years or longer. Some cases are transformed from the protracted course of acute viral hepatitis. Generally, chronic hepatitis can be divided into two types: chronic metastatic hepatitis and chronic active hepatitis.

Artemisia Capillaris Tea (*Yin Chen Hao Cha*)

Herba Artemisiae Capillaris (*Yin Chen Hao*)	100 grams
Peony root, *i.e.*, Radix Albus Paeoniae Lactiflorae (*Bai Shao*)	100 grams
Red dates, *i.e.*, Fructus Zizyphi Jujubae (*Da Zao*)	100 grams
Gardenia fruit, *i.e.*, Fructus Gardeniae Jasminoidis (*Shan Zhi Zi*)	50 grams
Radix Bupleuri (*Chai Hu*)	25 grams

65

Method of administration: Boil the above herbs in water. Discard the dregs and drink the liquid.

Functions: Courses the liver and disinhibits damp heat

Indications: This tea is suitable for the treatment or prevention of hepatitis during seasonal or epidemic outbreaks. During the season of infectious hepatitis, this herbal tea can be drunk as a beverage for prevention.

Isatis Root & Daqing Tea (*Ban Lan Gen Da Qing Cha*)

Radix Isatidis Seu Baphicacanthi (*Ban Lan Gen*)	30 grams
Folium Daqingye (*Da Qing Ye)*	30 grams
Tea leaves, *i.e.*, Folium Camelliae Theae (*Cha Ye*)	15 grams

Method of administration: Boil the above three ingredients with water and use the resulting liquid. Take 1 packet 2 times per day for 2 weeks.

Functions: Clears heat and resolves toxins, disinhibits dampness and abates jaundice

Indications: This tea is suitable for the treatment of acute hepatitis associated with damp heat and toxins.

Artemisia Capillaris & Plantain Tea (*Yin Chen Che Qian Cha*)

Plantain seeds, *i.e.*, Semen Plantaginis (*Che Qian Zi*)	300 grams
Herba Artemisiae Capillaris (*Yin Chen Hao*)	150 grams
Fresh willow leaves (*Xian Liu Ye*)	500 grams

Method of administration: Boil the above three ingredients with water. Use 1 packet for 2 days. This tea may be taken continually for half a month.

Functions: Clears heat and disinhibits dampness, benefits jaundice and abates yellowing

Indications: This tea is suitable for the treatment of acute hepatitis with jaundice due to damp heat. It is especially good for acute icteric hepatitis. One should take this tea in large doses.

Artemisia Tea (*Yin Chen Cha*)

Herba Artemisiae Capillaris (*Yin Chen Hao*)   30 grams
White sugar (*Bai Tang*)   Amount to taste

Method of administration: Decoct the artemisia capillaris with water, discard the dregs, and use the liquid. Add white sugar to the liquid and keep it in a thermos. Drink often, 1 packet per day at any time.

Functions: Clears heat, disinhibits dampness, and abates yellowing

Indications: This tea is suitable for the treatment of damp heat pattern icteric hepatitis.

Tumeric Clear the Liver Tea (*Yu Jin Qing Gan Cha*)

Vinegar stir-fried tumeric, *i.e.*, vinegar stir-fried Tuber
    Curcumae (*Cu Chao Yu Jin*)   10 grams
Mix-fried licorice root, *i.e.*, mix-fried Radix Glycyrrhizae Uralensis
    (*Zhi Gan Cao*)   5 grams
Green Tea, *i.e.*, Folium Camelliae Theae (*Lu Cha*)   2 grams
Honey (*Feng Mi*)   25 grams

Method of administration: Place the above four ingredients in a pot, add 1,000ml of water, and boil for 10 minutes. Strain and use the liquid. Drink often, 1 packet per day at any time.

Functions: Courses the liver and resolves depression, disinhibits dampness and dispels stasis

Indications: This tea is suitable for the treatment of hepatitis, cirrhosis of the liver, a fatty liver, and liver cancer exhibiting a liver depression/qi stagnation pattern.

Oldenlandia & Licorice Tea (*She She Gan Cao Cha*)

Herba Oldenlandiae Diffusae (*Bai Hua She She Cao*)	25 grams
Licorice root, *i.e.*, Radix Glycyrrhizae Uralensis (*Gan Cao*)	10 grams
Green Tea, *i.e.*, Folium Cameliae Theae (*Lu Cha*)	3 grams

Note: Use fresh oldenlandia if available.

Method of administration: Using gentle heat, boil the two herbs with just enough water to cover them. Decoct until 400ml are left. Strain the liquid and soak with the green Tea. Drink warm, 1 packet per day.

Functions: Clears heat and disinhibits dampness, scatters nodulation and resolves toxins

Indications: This tea is suitable for the treatment of hepatitis, cirrhosis of the liver, and liver cancer when exhibiting a pattern of dampness and heat.

Calm the Liver & Clear Heat Tea (*Ping Gan Qing Re Cha*)

Radix Gentianae Scabrae (*Long Dan Cao*)	1.8 grams
Vinegar-processed Radix Bupleuri (*Cu Zhi Chai Hu*)	1.8 grams
Radix Ligustici Wallichii (*Chuan Xiong*)	1.8 grams
Sweet chrysanthemum flower, *i.e.*, sweet Flos Chrysanthemi Morifolii (*Gan Ju Hua*)	3 grams
Uncooked Radix Rehmanniae (*Sheng Di*)	3 grams

Method of administration: Grind the above ingredients into a fine powder. Then boil with water. Take 1 packet per day.

Functions: Clears the liver and disinhibits the gallbladder

Indications: This tea is suitable for the treatment of hepatitis, cholecystitis, and acute conjunctivitis due to liver heat.

Aconite, Artemisia Capillaris & Ginger Tea (*Fu Zi Yin Jiang Cha*)

Radix Lateralis Praeparatus Aconiti Carmichaeli (*Zhi Fu Zi*)　　6 grams
Dry ginger, *i.e.*, dry Rhizoma Zingiberis (*Gan Jiang*)　　6 grams
Herba Artemisiae Capillaris (*Yin Chen Hao*)　　12 grams

Method of administration: Boil the herbs together with water. Drink as a tea.

Functions: Scatters cold, dispels damp, and abates yellowing

Indications: This tea is suitable for the treatment of yin jaundice due to conversion from yang jaundice after a long period of time. It may also be due to devitalized spleen yang or brewing of cold and dampness causing the body and eyes to be a darkish, sallow yellow. This is accompanied by lassitude of the spirit, fatigue, lack of strength, cold limbs, and short voidings of scant urine.

Contraindications: Prepared aconite is contraindicated during pregnancy.

Day Lily Protect the Liver Tea (*Huang Hua Bao Gan Cha*)

Day lily flowers, *i.e.*, Flos Hemerocallis (*Huang Hua Cai*)　　10 grams
Fresh licorice root, *i.e.*, uncooked Radix Glycyrrhizae Uralensis
　(*Sheng Gan Cao*)　　8 grams
Fructus Schisandrae Chinensis (*Wu Wei Zi*)　　5 grams
Red dates, *i.e.*, Fructus Zizyphi Jujubae (*Da Zao*)　　50 grams

Method of administration: Rinse the above herbs well and soak them in boiling water in a large cup for 5 minutes. Strain and drink the liquid. Use 1 packet per day. This tea may be taken frequently.

Functions: Clears heat and disinhibits dampness, nourishes the blood and supplements the liver

Indications: This tea is suitable for the treatment of hepatitis B, chronic active hepatitis (CAH), and icteric hepatitis. This is a good formula for individuals with hepatitis to drink as a beverage. It helps to stabilize and improve the condition.

Cholecystitis Teas

Cholecystitis can be divided into acute and chronic types. Acute cholecystitis may be due to bacterial infection, chemical irritants, gallstones, highly concentrated bile, or pancreatic reflux into the gallbladder. Its common clinical signs are fever, pain in the right upper abdomen, compression pain, vomiting, and increased white blood cells. Jaundice is visible in 25% of patients. The symptoms of chronic cholecystitis are less severe than the acute form but are recurring. Chronic cholecystitis without gallstones is rare. The following medicinal tea formula should be chosen based on the individual's pattern discrimination and their signs and symptoms. With chronic cholecystitis, diet is extremely important as is stress reduction and relaxation.

Jinqian, Patrinia & Artemisia Capillaris Tea
(*Jin Qian Bai Jiang Yin Chen Cha*)

Herba Jinqiancao (*Jin Qian Cao*)	30 grams
Herba Patriniae Heterophyllae Cum Radice (*Bai Jiang Cao*)	30 grams
Herba Artemisiae Capillaris (*Yin Chen Hao*)	30 grams
White sugar (*Bai Tang*)	Amount to taste

Method of administration: Boil the three herbs with water, strain, and reserve the liquid. Add the white sugar to the liquid and dissolve. Use 1 packet per day. This tea should be drunk warm.

Functions: Disinhibits the gallbladder, expels stones, and disperses inflammation

Indications: This tea is suitable for the treatment of chronic cholecystitis and cholelithiasis. For best results, it should be drunk quite often.

Corn Silk Tea (*Yu Mi Xu Cha*)

Corn silk, *i.e.*, Stylus Zeae Maydis (*Yu Mi Xu*)   A suitable amount

Method of administration: Place the corn silk into a pot, add water, and boil briefly. Drink the resulting tea frequently.

Functions: Discharges heat and disinhibits urination, disinhibits the gallbladder and calms the liver

Indications: This tea is suitable for the treatment of cholecystitis, gallstones, diabetes, hypertension, and nephritic edema due to accumulation of dampness internally.

Contraindications: Alcohol, glutinous, sweet or sticky rice, fish roe, dry roe, fatty meats, and pungent, hot, and bitter foods should not be eaten while taking this tea. Actually, none of these foods should be eaten by anyone with cholecystitis due to dampness and heat.

Disperse Inflammation & Disinhibit the Gallbladder Tea (*Xiao Yan Li Dan Cha*)

Dandelion, *i.e.*, Herba Taraxaci Mongolici Cum Radice (*Pu Gong Ying*) 30 grams
Herba Artemisiae Capillaris (*Yin Chen Hao*)   30 grams
Corn silk, *i.e.*, Stylus Zeae Maydis (*Yu Mi Xu*)   30 grams

71

White sugar (*Bai Tang*)   Amount to taste

Method of administration: Boil the herbs in 1,000ml water and cook until 750ml remains. Strain and use the liquid. Add the white sugar and drink warm. Use 1 packet per day taken in 3 divided doses of 250ml each.

Functions: Clears heat and disinhibits dampness, disperses inflammation and disinhibits the gallbladder

Indications: This tea is suitable for the treatment of cholecystitis and icteric hepatitis due to dampness and heat.

Nephritis Teas

Nephritis is divided into two types: acute and chronic. Acute nephritis is a type of inflammatory condition due to bacteria or their toxins, such as beta hemolytic streptococcus, septicemia, or toxic compounds. Clinically, its main symptoms are generalized edema, oliguria, hematuria, and proteinuria. It can also raise the blood pressure. Chronic nephritis is an inflammatory condition which is more progressive. The course of chronic nephritis is longer. Its main symptoms based on routine urine examination are proteinuria, bloody hyaline, and granular casts on microscopic exam. These are accompanied by edema, high blood pressure, and varying degrees of kidney damage. In TCM, nephritis belongs to the category of "water swelling."

Imperata Tea (*Mao Gen Cha*)

Rhizoma Imperatae Cylindricae (*Bai Mao Gen*)   10 grams
Tea leaves, *i.e.*, Folium Camelliae Theae (*Cha Ye*)   5 grams

Method of administration: Pick out the root and tassel of the imperata and wash it well. Boil the herb and Tea leaves with water. Drink the liquid. Use 1 packet per day taken at any time.

72

Functions: Clears heat and disinhibits the urine, disperses inflammation and resolves toxins, cools the blood and stops bleeding

Indications: This tea is suitable for the treatment of acute and chronic nephritis, edema, acute infectious hepatitis, and hematuria due to dampness and heat.

Corn Silk Disperse Swelling Tea (*Yu Mi Xu Xiao Zhong Cha*)

Corn silk, *i.e.*, Stylus Zeae Maydis (*Yu Mi Xu*)	50 grams
Watermelon peel, *i.e.*, Exocarpium Citrulli Vulgaris (*Xi Gua Pi*)	50 grams
Aduki beans, *i.e.*, Semen Phaseoli Calcarati (*Chi Xiao Dou*)	50 grams

Note: Aduki beans are small red beans, not the larger kidney beans. They are also sold sometimes in the West under the name azuki beans. Both names are originally Japanese.

Method of administration: Wash the herbs well. Place them in a pot, add water, and boil. Use 1 packet per day. Strain off the liquid and drink it as a tea.

Functions: Disinhibits the urine and disperses swelling

Indications: This tea is suitable for the treatment of nephritic water swelling. In particular, it treats damp heat patterns of acute and chronic nephritis.

Plantain Tea (*Che Qian Cao Cha*)

Plantain leaves, *i.e.*, Herba Plantaginis (*Che Qian Cao*)	20 grams

Method of administration: Grind the herb into a coarse powder. Boil with water or soak in boiling water. Use 1 packet per day. Drink this freely as a tea.

Functions: Clears damp heat and disinhibits the urine

Indications: This tea is suitable for the treatment of nephritic water swelling, chronic pyelonephritis, cystitis, dribbling urinary block, and hypertension.

Watermelon & Imperata Tea (*Xi Gua Bai Mao Cha*)

Watermelon peel, *i.e.*, Exocarpium Citrulli Vulgaris (*Xi Gua Pi*)   60 grams
Fresh Rhizoma Imperatae Cylindricae (*Xian Bai Mao Gen*)   90 grams

Method of administration: Boil these two ingredients together, remove the dregs, and drink the liquid. Use 1 packet per day taken in 3 divided doses.

Functions: Clears heat, cools the blood, and disinhibits the urine

Indications: This tea is suitable for the treatment of chronic nephritis, hematuria, casts in the urine, edema, and hypertension. This formula also works for acute nephritic water swelling.

Lotus Seed & Brown Sugar Tea (*Lian Zi Hong Tang Cha*)

Lotus seeds, *i.e.*, Semen Nelumbinis Nuciferae (*Lian Zi*)   50 grams
Tea leaves, *i.e.*, Folium Camelliae Theae (*Cha Ye*)   3 grams
Brown sugar (*Hong Tang*)   30 grams

Method of administration: Prepare the Tea and set aside. Soak the lotus seeds in warm water for 5 hours. Then remove and place in a pot. Add the brown sugar and water. Then cook thoroughly. Finally, add the Tea water. Use 1 packet per day. Drink this freely as a tea.

Functions: Nourishes the heart and fortifies the spleen, boosts the kidneys and secures the essence

Indications: This tea is suitable for the treatment of nephritic water swelling. It is also beneficial for nephritic water swelling with blood stasis. However, it is only effective when used consistently.

Nourish the Kidneys Tea (*Yang Shen Cha*)

Radix Astragali Membranacei (*Huang Qi*)	15 grams
Radix Salviae Miltiorrhizae (*Dan Shen*)	10 grams
Hawthorn fruit, *i.e.*, Fructus Crataegi (*Shan Zha*)	10 grams

Method of administration: Place the above three ingredients in a cup and soak the herbs in boiling water. Drink 1 cup approximately 1 hour before sleep.

Functions: Quickens the blood and transforms stasis

Indications: This tea is suitable for the treatment of chronic nephritis with low-grade renal failure exhibiting a pattern of blood stasis. For instance, there may be a purplish tongue or static spots or macules on the tongue and a wiry and/or choppy pulse.

Strangury Teas

The main symptom of strangurious conditions is urinary irritation. Strangurious conditions refers to frequent, short, inhibited voidings of urine, dribbling urine with sharp pain, an urge to urinate without success, tension in the lower abdomen, pain that reaches up to umbilicus, and an inhibited urinary tract. In Western medicine, pyelonephritis, cystitis, urethritis, urinary stone, and renal tuberculosis all belong to the category of strangurious conditions. Herbal tea formulas have a good result on these conditions when prescribed based on a TCM pattern discrimination.

Lophatherum & Plantain Tea (*Zhu Ye Che Qian Cha*)

Plantain leaf, *i.e.*, Herba Plantaginis (*Che Qian Cao*)	100 grams
Herba Lophatheri Gracilis (*Dan Zhu Ye*)	10 grams
Uncooked licorice root, *i.e.*, uncooked Radix Glycyrrhizae Uralensis (*Sheng Gan Cao*)	10 grams
White sugar (*Bai Tang*)	Amount to taste

Method of administration: Boil the above four ingredients, remove the dregs, and reserve the liquid. Drink 1 packet per day.

Functions: Clears and disinhibits dampness and heat

Indications: This tea is suitable for the treatment of cystitis and urethritis with short, painful, inhibited voidings of urine due to damp heat pouring down to the bladder.

Contraindications: This formula should not be taken for a long period of time or it will damage yin fluids and stomach qi.

Pyrrosia Tea (*Shi Wei Cha*)

Folium Pyrrosiae (*Shi Wei*)	60 grams
Plantain leaf, *i.e.*, Herba Plantaginis (*Che Qian Cao*)	60 grams
Gardenia fruit, *i.e.*, Fructus Gardeniae Jasminoidis (*Shan Zhi Zi*)	30 grams
Licorice root, *i.e.*, Radix Glycyrrhizae Uralensis (*Gan Cao*)	15 grams

Method of administration: Grind the above herbs into a coarse powder. Boil the resulting powder in water. Use 1 packet per day. This tea may be drunk frequently.

Functions: Disinhibits the urine and expels stones

Indications: This tea is suitable for the treatment of pyelonephritis, cystitis, and urinary stones due to dampness and heat.

Tetrapanax Tea (*Tong Cao Cha*)

Medulla Tetrapanacis Papyriferi (*Tong Cao*)	3 grams
Medulla Junci Effusi (*Deng Xin Cao*)	3 grams
Green Tea, *i.e.*, Folium Camelliae Theae (*Lu Cha*)	6 grams
Rhizoma Imperatae Cylindricae (*Bai Mao Gen*)	30 grams

Method of administration: Soak the above ingredients in boiling water. Use 1 packet per day. Drink this freely throughout the day as a tea.

Functions: Clears heat, disinhibits the urine, and frees strangurious conditions

Indications: This tea is suitable for the treatment of acute urinary tract infection with obstructed, dribbling urine due to damp heat.

Eclipta Tea (*Han Lian Cao Cha*)

Herba Ecliptae Prostratae (*Han Lian Cao*)	20 grams
Plantain leaf, *i.e.*, Herba Plantaginis (*Che Qian Cao*)	20 grams
White sugar (*Bai Tang*)	Amount to taste

Method of administration: Grind the herbs into a coarse powder, boil with water, strain, and save the liquid. Add the sugar to the liquid and drink after the sugar has dissolved.

Functions: Clears heat and disinhibits the urination, cools the blood and stops bleeding

Indications: This tea is suitable for the treatment of patients with hematuria due to dampness and heat. In this case, heat is causing the blood to move recklessly or frenetically outside its pathways.

Urinary Tract Stone Teas

Urinary tract stones include kidney stones (renal calculi), stones in the ureters (urinary calculi), or stones in the bladder (vesicular calculi). In TCM, these belong to the categories of sand strangury, stone strangury, and blood strangury. The main symptoms are gripping pain in the low back and abdominal areas, hematuria, and difficult urination. In Western medicine, the causes of the urinary tract stones are relatively complicated and, in some cases, unknown. Nevertheless, they do have a close relationship with environmental factors, such as dehydration in arid climates, general debility, and urinary system disease. In TCM, urinary tract stones are usually believed to be due to damp heat brewing and binding in the low burner or boiling, stewing, and inhibited qi transformation.

Expelling Stones Tea (*Pai Shi Cha*)

Herba Jinqiancao (*Jin Qian Cao*)	50 grams
Spora Lygodii Japonici (*Hai Jin Sha*)	15 grams

Method of administration: Boil the above two herbs in water. Discard the dregs and use the liquid. Drink frequently as a beverage. Use 1 packet per day.

Functions: Clears heat and dispels dampness, disinhibits the urine and frees strangury

Indications: This tea is suitable for the treatment of urinary tract stones, gallbladder stones (cholecystolithiasis), urinary tract infection, and nephritic edema due to damp heat.

Lygodium Tea (*Hai Jin Sha Cha*)

Spora Lygodii Japonici (*Hai Jin Sha*)	15 grams
Green Tea, *i.e.*, Folium Camelliae Theae (*Lu Cha*)	2 grams

Method of administration: Place the two ingredients in a cup and steep in boiling water. Cover for 5 minutes. Use 1 packet per day. Each day upon arising, drink 1 cup while the stomach is still empty. During the day, it can be taken at any time. Use for 2 months for a complete treatment.

Functions: Clears heat and percolates dampness, disinhibits the urine and frees strangury, downbears fire and resolves toxins

Indications: This tea is suitable for the treatment of kidney stones, bladder stones, inhibited urination, hot and painful urine, and yellow and red urine all due to damp heat. The tongue coating is yellow and slimy.

Water Chestnut & Chicken Gizzard Tea (*Bi Qi Nei Jin Cha*)

Water chestnut, *i.e.*, Tuber Eleocharis Dulcis (*Bi Qi*)	120 grams
Chicken gizzard lining, *i.e.*, Endothelium Corneum Gigeriae Galli (*Ji Nei Jin*)	15 grams

Method of administration: Boil the above two ingredients together. Discard the dregs and drink the liquid. Use 1 packet per day. Drink this freely as a tea.

Functions: Clears heat and transforms stones

Indications: This tea is suitable for the treatment of stone strangury, occasional sand and stone in the urine, yellow, reddish, and turbid urine, difficult and astringent urination with burning pain, occasional sudden obstruction to the urine, urgency to urinate, sharp pain in the urinary tract, or unbearable abdominal and/or low back pain or blood appearing in the urine.

Three Golds Tea (*San Jin Cha*)

Herba Jinqiancao (*Jin Qian Cao*)	10 grams
Spora Lygodii Japonici (*Hai Jin Sha*)	10 grams
Chicken gizzard lining, *i.e.*, Endothelium Corneum Gigeriae Galli (*Ji Nei Jin*)	15 grams

Note: All three of these medicinals have the word *jin* or gold in their name. Hence the name of the formula, "Three Golds Tea."

Method of administration: Wrap the spora lygodii in cloth and boil it with the other two herbs. Discard the dregs and drink the liquid. Use 1 packet per day. Drink this frequently as a tea.

Functions: Clears heat and expels stones

Indications: This tea is suitable for the treatment of stone strangury. This refers to occasional sand and stones in the urine, yellow, reddish, and turbid urine, difficult and astringent urination with burning pain, occasional, sudden obstruction to the urine, urgency to urinate, sharp pain in the urinary tract, or unbearable abdominal and/or low back pain or blood appearing in the urine. The tongue is predominantly red with a thin, yellow coating. The pulse is slightly rapid.

Jinqiancao & Corn Silk Tea (*Qian Cao Yu Mi Cha*)

Herba Jinqiancao (*Jin Qian Cao*)	30-60 grams
Corn silk, *i.e.*, Stylus Zeae Maydis (*Yu Mi Xu*)	30-60 grams
Green Tea, *i.e.*, Folium Cameliae Theae (*Lu Cha*)	5 grams

Method of administration: Place these three ingredients in a pot and add enough water to cover the herbs. Boil for 10-15 minutes. Boil twice and combine the liquids from these two boilings together. Another method is to grind these three ingredients into a coarse powder. Place this powder into a teapot and soak in boiling water for 20 minutes. Use 1 packet per day and drink it frequently at any time.

Functions: Clears heat and transforms dampness, disinhibits the urine and resolves stones

Indications: This tea is suitable for the treatment of stones in the urinary tract, kidney stones, and gallstones due to damp heat.

Walnut Tea (*Hu Tao Cha*)

Walnut, *i.e.*, Semen Juglandis Regiae (*Hu Tao Ren*)	90 grams
White sugar (*Bai Tang*)	90 grams

Method of administration: Grind the shelled walnuts into a powder, add water, and then mix into a milky paste. Pour into a pot, add 500 grams of water, and the sugar. Mix well and bring the mixture to a boil. Take 1 packet per day and drink it all at once.

Functions: Frees strangury and disperses stones

Indications: This tea is suitable for the treatment of stones in different parts of the urinary tract system. This is based on empirical experience, not on TCM theory. Usually, a milky urine is expelled along with the stones after several days administration.

Shan Qi Teas

Shan qi, also called qi egg in TCM, refers to hernias. Hernias are protrusions or projections of a part of an organ through the wall of the cavity that normally contains it. Inguinal hernias, which account for 90% of all hernias, are protrusions of a section of the intestines. They may descend into the scrotum, causing swelling, distention, and pain.

Fennel Tea (*Hui Xiang Cha*)

Fennel seeds, *i.e.,* Fructus Foeniculi Vulgaris (*Xiao Hui Xiang*)   9-15 grams

Method of administration: Wrap this herb in clean cotton gauze and place in a cup. Steep in boiling water and drink as a tea.

Functions: Rectifies the qi and stops pain

Indications: This tea is suitable for the treatment of incarcerated hernia—the more acute the condition, the better the results. After drinking, one should lie on their back with their knees bent. Usually the symptoms will be reduced in 1/2 hour. In terms of TCM pattern, this tea is specifically for a hernia characterized as a cold stagnation in the liver channel pattern.

Contraindications: If the *shan* qi incarceration becomes chronic, there is the possibility of necrosis and perforation. In that case, one should not attempt to use this formula. Such conditions require surgical repair.

Leechee & Olive Tea (*Li Gan Cha*)

Leechee nut, *i.e.*, Semen Litchi Chinensis (*Li Zhi He*)   10 grams
Chinese olive pit, *i.e.*, Semen Canarii (*Gan Lan He*)   10 grams

Method of administration: Break these ingredients into pieces by pounding and then steep in boiling water. Drink frequently as a tea.

Functions: Rectifies the qi and scatters nodulation, stops pain

Indications: This tea is suitable for the treatment of cold *shan*.

Olive & Pomegranate Tea (*Qing Guo Shi Liu Cha*)

Chinese olive, *i.e.*, Fructus Canarii (*Gan Lan*)   5-10 grams
Pomegranate skin, *i.e.*, Pericarpium Punicae Granati (*Shi Liu Pi*)   5-10 grams

Method of administration: Cut the olives into slices and tear the pomegranate skin into pieces. Place these in a cup and soak in boiling water. Drink the resulting liquid as a tea.

Functions: Clears heat and astringes the intestines

Indications: This tea is suitable for the treatment of *shan* qi due to loss of astringency, not due to cold stagnation.

A Pair of Pits Tea (*Shuang He Cha*)

Leechee nut, *i.e.*, Semen Litchi Chinensis (*Li Zhi He*)   10-15 grams

Tangerine seeds, *i.e.*, Semen Citri Reticulatae (*Ju He*)   10-15 grams
Brown sugar (*Hong Tang*)   Amount to taste

Method of administration: Boil the herbs in water, discard the dregs, and drink the liquid. When drinking, brown sugar may be added to taste. Drink warm as a tea.

Functions: Moves the qi and scatters cold, scatters nodulation and stops pain

Indications: This tea is suitable for the treatment of *shan qi* pain due to cold stagnating in the liver channel.

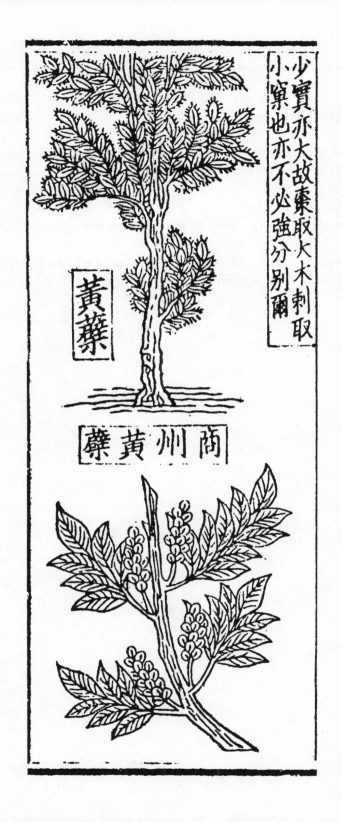

少實亦大故棗取火木刺取
小棘也亦不必強分別爾

黃蘗

商州黃蘗

4
Cardiovascular Diseases

Hypertension Teas

Hypertension refers to arterial blood pressure which is higher than normal. In general, if the systolic pressure is above 140mm of mercury or the diastolic pressure is above 90mm mercury, the individual is considered to have an elevated blood pressure. There are a number of causes of high blood pressure and high blood pressure can accompany various other diseases. Hypertension is sometimes called the silent killer because it may have no symptoms. In more severe cases, there may be dizziness, headache, tinnitus, blurred vision, palpitations, and irritability. In TCM, hypertension is related to an imbalance of yin and yang, and the disease primarily involves the liver and kidneys. The typical patterns associated with hypertension are hyperactivity of liver yang, kidney yin vacuity, and kidney yin and yang vacuity. Complications may then include liver wind, static blood, and phlegm turbidity. Clinically, hypertension is often seen as a combination of vacuity and repletion. Chinese medicinal teas for hypertension should be chosen on the basis of a TCM pattern discrimination, taking into account all of a person's signs and symptoms.

Chrysanthemum Flower & Hawthorn Tea (*Ju Hua Shan Zha Cha*)

Chrysanthemum flower, *i.e.*, Flos Chrysanthemi Morifolii (*Ju Hua*)	10 grams
Tea leaves, *i.e.*, Folium Cameliae Theae (*Cha Ye*)	10 grams
Hawthorn fruit, *i.e.*, Fructus Crataegi (*Shan Zha*)	30 grams

Method of administration: Place these ingredients in a cup. Pour in boiling water and let steep. Use 1 packet per day. Drink this freely as a tea.

Functions: Clears heat and downbears phlegm, disperses food and fortifies the stomach, lowers lipids

Indications: This tea is suitable for the treatment of hypertension, coronary heart disease, and high cholesterol associated with liver yang hyperactivity or liver fire patterns.

Gardenia Fruit Tea (*Zhi Zi Cha*)

Young Tea leaves, *i.e.* young Folium Cameliae Theae (*Ya Cha*)   30 grams
Gardenia fruit, *i.e.*, Fructus Gardeniae Jasminoidis (*Shan Zhi Zi*)   30 grams

Method of administration: Pour 800-1,000ml of water into a pot containing the above two ingredients. Boil the herbs into a strong liquid or until approximately 400-500ml of liquid are left. Drink warm. Use 1 packet per day taken in two divided doses, once in the morning and once in the afternoon.

Functions: Drains fire and clears the liver, cools the blood and downbears pressure

Indications: This tea is suitable for the treatment of hypertension with headache and dizziness due to liver yang hyperactivity and liver fire.

Hawthorn & Two Flowers Tea (*Shan Zha Er Hua Cha*)

Hawthorn fruit, *i.e.*, Fructus Crataegi (*Shan Zha*)   25 grams
Honeysuckle flower, *i.e.*, Flos Lonicerae Japonicae (*Jin Yin Hua*)   25 grams
Chrysanthemum flower, *i.e.*, Flos Chrysanthemi Morifolii (*Ju Hua*)   25 grams

Method of administration: Place the above three ingredients in a large cup. Pour in boiling water, cover for a short time, and then drink. Use 1 packet per day. Drink this freely as a tea.

Functions: Fortifies the spleen, clears heat, and lowers lipids

Indications: This tea is suitable for the treatment of hypertension and high cholesterol due to liver heat and spleen vacuity.

Chrysanthemum, Hawthorn & Cassia Tea (*Ju Zha Jue Ming Cha*)

Chrysanthemum flower, *i.e.*, Flos Chrysanthemi Morifolii (*Ju Hua*) 8 grams
Uncooked hawthorn fruit slices, *i.e.*, uncooked Fructus Crataegi
(*Sheng Shan Zha Pian*)   15 grams
Semen Cassiae Torae (*Jue Ming Zi*)   15 grams

Method of administration: Place the above three ingredients into a thermal cup, pour in boiling water, and steep. Cover the cup tightly for 30 minutes and then drink the resulting tea. Use 1 packet per day. Drink this freely as a tea.

Functions: Courses wind and resolves toxins, clears the liver, downbears pressure, and disperses food stagnation

Indications: This tea is suitable for the treatment of hypertension and coronary heart disease due to liver yang hyperactivity and liver fire.

Chrysanthemum & Sophora Tea (*Ju Huai Cha*)

Chrysanthemum flower, *i.e.*, Flos Chrysanthemi Morifolii (*Ju Hua*) 3 grams
Flos Immaturus Sophorae Japonicae (*Huai Hua Mi*)   3 grams
Green Tea, *i.e.*, Folium Cameliae Theae (*Lu Cha*)   3 grams

Method of administration: Place the above three ingredients in a cup. Pour in boiling water, cover tightly, and let soak for 5 minutes. Use 1 packet per day. Drink this freely as a tea.

Functions: Calms the liver and dispels wind, clears fire and downbears pressure

Indications: This tea is suitable for the treatment of headache caused by hypertension and the sensation of pressure in the head with dizziness due to liver yang hyperactivity.

Chrysanthemum & Cassia Downbear Pressure Tea (*Ju Ming Jiang Ya Cha*)

White chrysanthemum flower, *i.e.*, Flos Chrysanthemi Morifolii
    (*Bai Ju Hua*)   10 grams
Semen Cassiae Torae (*Jue Ming Zi*)   15 grams

Method of administration: Place these two ingredients in a cup, pour in boiling water, and let soak. Use 1 packet per day. Drink this freely as a tea.

Functions: Clears the liver and downbears pressure, moistens the intestines and frees the stools

Indications: This tea is suitable for the treatment of hypertension due to liver yang hyperactivity with habitual constipation.

Prunella Downbear Pressure Tea (*Xia Ku Cao Jiang Ya Cha*)

Selfheal spike, *i.e.*, Spica Prunellae Vulgaris (*Xia Ku Cao*)   10 grams
Plantain leaf, *i.e.*, Herba Plantaginis (*Che Qian Cao*)   12 grams

Method of administration: Wash the selfheal spikes and plantain leaves and then place them in a cup. Pour in boiling water and let soak. Use 1 packet per day. Drink freely as a tea.

Functions: Clears heat, disinhibits water, and downbears pressure

Indications: This tea is suitable for hypertension with dizziness and headache due to liver yang hyperactivity. It can be taken daily by individuals with hypertension. However, the blood pressure needs to be monitored regularly in order to prevent symptoms of low blood pressure. Since this tea functions, in part, as a diuretic, persons using this tea should be careful of their potassium levels.

Three Treasures Tea (*San Bao Cha*)

Chrysanthemum flower, *i.e.*, Flos Chrysanthemi Morifolii (*Ju Hua*)   6 grams
Arhat fruit, *i.e.*, Fructus Mormordicae Grosvenori (*Luo Han Guo*)   6 grams
Pu Er Tea, *i.e.*, Pu Er Folium Cameliae Theae (*Pu Er Cha*)   6 grams

Note: Pu Er Tea is a particular type of Tea from Yunnan province. In China, different types of Tea grown in different regions are processed in slightly different ways and are believed to have different medicinal values and uses.

Method of administration: Grind the above three herbs into a coarse powder and place inside paper filter bags (18 grams in each bag). Pour boiling water over the bag and allow to steep. Use 1 packet per day and drink freely as a tea.

Functions: Downbears pressure, disperses lipids, and reduces obesity

Indications: This tea may be used for the prevention and treatment of hypertension and high cholesterol as well as headache and dizziness caused by liver yang hyperactivity.

Hypotension Teas

Hypotension refers to below normal systolic and diastolic blood pressures. If the systolic and diastolic pressures are at or below 90mm Hg and 60mm Hg respectively, this is considered hypotension. Hypotension may be due to hemorrhage, anemia, infection, fever, debilitating or wasting diseases, adrenal insufficiency, or, in acute instances, to shock and collapse. The main symptoms of hypotension are frequent dizziness, headache, head clouding, a tendency to fatigue, cool extremities, and a relaxed, slow pulse. Dizziness may only occur on standing up rapidly. This is referred to as orthostatic hypotension. In TCM, this condition is dealt with under the categories of "dizziness" and "headache."

It is usually due to vacuity and its treatment, therefore, focuses primarily on supplementing. In Western medicine, hypotension is not always considered a disease. In Chinese medicine, hypotension is considered a disease and is treated in order to bring the blood pressure up to normal. In doing this, the patient typically experiences more energy and warmer hands and feet.

Licorice & Red Dates Tea (*Gan Cao Cha*)

Uncooked licorice root, *i.e.*, uncooked Radix Glycyrrhizae Uralensis (*Sheng Gan Cao*)	10 grams
Red dates, *i.e.*, Fructus Zizyphi Jujubae (*Da Zao*)	20 grams

Method of administration: Steep these two herbs in boiling water, cover for 15 minutes, and then drink. Use 1 packet per day.

Functions: Fortifies the spleen, disperses summerheat, and prevents disease

Indications: This tea is suitable for the treatment of hypotension due to heart and spleen qi vacuity, dry, itchy throat, and troubled sleep due to heart vacuity.

Note: Licorice can raise the blood pressure as this simple tea suggests. Therefore, patient's with high blood pressure should not take teas which contain licorice or, if they do, their blood pressure should be monitored regularly.

Contraindications: Patients with average constitution and health should not take this formula to prevent disease. It should only be used for that purpose by people with a weak bodily constitution.

Double Cinnamon Tea (*Shuang Gui Cha*)

Cinnamon twig, *i.e.*, Ramulus Cinnamomi Cassiae (*Gui Zhi*)	15 grams
Cinnamon bark, *i.e.*, Cortex Cinnamomi Cassiae (*Rou Gui*)	15 grams
Mixed-fried licorice root, *i.e.*, mix-fried Radix Glycyrrhizae	

Uralensis (*Zhi Gan Cao*)   15 grams

Method of administration: Place these three herbs in a pot, add water, and boil briefly. Another method is to rinse the herbs well, place in a cup, and steep in boiling water. Drink this frequently as a tea, 1 packet per day.

Functions: Warms yang and increases pressure

Indications: This tea is suitable for the treatment of excessively low blood pressure due to yang vacuity with fear of cold, cold limbs, dizziness, lack of strength, and a deep, slow pulse.

Coronary Heart Disease Teas

Coronary heart disease is a shortened name for coronary atherosclerotic cardiopathy. It is common among the middle-aged and elderly. Its primary symptoms are typically pain or a sensation of compression in the chest that occurs suddenly and generally lasts 3-5 minutes per episode. This is often accompanied by a drained white facial complexion, horrified spirit-affect, chest oppression and stifling qi, difficult breathing, and a cold sweat. This disease belongs to the categories of "chest bi" and "heart pain" in TCM. Treatment should be based on the principle, "In an acute condition, treat the branch; in chronic cases, treat the root." During the painful period, the focus should be on freeing the flow and quickening the blood, transforming stasis, rectifying the qi, and freeing yang. When the pain is alleviated, the treatment should focus on regulating the viscera and bowels, qi and blood, and banking up and supplementing the righteous qi.

Hawthorn & Motherwort Tea (*Shan Zha Yi Mu Cha*)

Hawthorn fruit, *i.e.*, Fructus Crataegi (*Shan Zha*)   30 grams
Motherwort, *i.e.*, Herba Leonuri Heterophylli (*Yi Mu Cao*)   10 grams
Tea, *i.e.*, Folium Camelliae Theae (*Cha*)   5 grams

Method of administration: Place these three ingredients in a cup and pour in boiling water. Drink this daily as a tea.

Functions: Clears heat and transforms phlegm, quickens the blood, lowers lipids, and frees the network vessels

Indications: This tea is suitable for the treatment of coronary disease and high cholesterol associated with a pattern of blood stasis.

Salvia Tea (*Dan Shen Cha*)

Radix Salviae Miltiorrhizae (*Dan Shen*)   9 grams
Green Tea, *i.e.*, Folium Camelliae Theae (*Lu Cha*)   3 grams

Method of administration: Grind the root into a coarse powder. Steep this powder and the Tea in boiling water for 10 minutes. Drink 1 packet per day at any time.

Functions: Quickens the blood and transforms stasis, stops pain and eliminates vexation

Indications: This tea is suitable for the treatment of coronary heart disease and for the prevention of angina pectoris associated with a pattern of blood stasis. This formula is also suitable for the treatment and prevention of high cholesterol if there are symptoms of blood stasis.

Hawthorn, Chrysanthemum & Cassia Tea (*Zha Ju Jue Ming Cha*)

Chrysanthemum flower, *i.e.*, Flos Chrysanthemi Morifolii (*Ju Hua*)   5 grams
Uncooked hawthorn fruit, *i.e.*, uncooked Fructus Crataegi
   (*Sheng Shan Zha*)   10 grams
Semen Cassiae Torae (*Jue Ming Zi*)   15 grams

Method of administration: Rinse the herbs well and boil in a pot with water for 20 minutes. Another method is to steep the herbs in a thermos, covered in boiling water for 30 minutes. Use 1 packet per day. Drink this frequently at any time.

Functions: Calms the liver, clears heat, and quickens the blood

Indications: This tea is suitable for coronary heart disease, angina pectoris, and hypertension. This tea can also prevent and treat angiocardiopathy. And it can be taken daily as a tea for individuals with coronary disease.

Salvia & (Hawthorn) Fruit Tea (*Shen Guo Cha*)

Radix Salviae Miltiorrhizae (*Dan Shen*)	10 grams
Uncooked hawthorn fruit (sliced), *i.e.*, uncooked Fructus Crataegi (*Sheng Shan Zha Pian*)	10 grams
Tuber Ophiopogonis Japonici (*Mai Men Dong*)	5 grams

Method of administration: Place these herbs in a cup, add boiling water, cover, and soak for 30 minutes. Drink warm. It may be taken frequently.

Functions: Quickens the blood and transforms stasis

Indications: This tea is suitable for preventing and treating coronary heart disease and hypertension due to blood stasis. It can soften sclerotic blood vessels.

Rheumatic Heart Disease Tea

Rheumatic heart disease is due to the repeated occurrence of rheumatic endocarditis. This leaves scaring and adhesions on the cardiac valves which result in valve deformation (valvular inadequacy or stenosis), thus causing obstruction of blood flow, cardiac murmur, increased heart burden, enlargement of the heart, and even heart failure. This usually occurs between the ages of 20-40, more commonly in women. Approximately half of the patients do not have any obvious history of rheumatic disease. Its main signs are dyspnea and water swelling or edema. In TCM, this disease belongs to the categories of "racing of the heart" and "water swelling." Treatment focuses on boosting the qi and nourishing the heart, warming yang and disinhibiting water, and quickening the blood and transforming stasis.

Sunflower Plate Tea (*Kui Pan Cha*)

Sunflower plate, *i.e.*, the dried seedless head of the large Sunflower (*Kui Pan*)	1 head

Method of administration: Cut the sunflower plate into four pieces. Boil 1 piece each time with water for 1 dose. Drink warm at any time, 2 doses per day.

Functions: Dispels wind and dampness, tranquilizes the heart spirit

Indications: This tea is suitable for rheumatic mitral stenosis, chest oppression, palpitations, and irregular heart beat.

Palpitation Teas

Palpitations refers to a rapid, violent throbbing or fluttering of the heart that is perceptible to the individual. There may also be feelings of fright. This is often seen along with symptoms such as insomnia, impaired memory, dizziness, and tinnitus. They may occur due to emotional changes, such as anxiety, or with excessive exhaustion. In Western medicine, they may either be a symptom of neurosis or different types of heart diseases with arrhythmias. In TCM, they are included under "fright palpitations" and "racing of the heart."

Sour Dates & Euryales Tea (*Suan Zao Qian Shi Cha*)

Longan fruit, *i.e.*, Arillus Euphoriae Longanae (*Long Yan Rou*)	10 grams
Stir-fried Semen Ziziphi Spinosae (*Chao Suan Zao Ren*)	10 grams
Semen Euryalis Ferocis (*Qian Shi*)	12 grams

Method of administration: Place these herbs in a pot, add water, and boil over a gentle fire. Discard the dregs and save the liquid. Use 1 packet per day and take continuously for 15 days. This equals 1 course of treatment.

Functions: Nourishes the blood and quiets the spirit, boosts the kidneys and secures essence

Indications: This tea is suitable for the treatment of palpitations, racing of the heart, insomnia, lassitude of the spirit, and fatigue due to a heart and kidney vacuity. This formula secures the root, reduces expenditure, supplements vacuity, and supports the righteous.

Contraindications: This tea is contraindicated in individuals suffering from a common cold.

Biota Seed Tea (*Bai Zi Ren Cha*)

Stir-fried Semen Biotae Orientalis (*Chao Bai Zi Ren*)   15 grams

Method of administration: Pick out the impurities and eliminate the remaining shells and skin of the biota seeds. Lightly pound the stir-fried biota seeds into pieces. Use 10-15 grams each time, placing them in a cup and steeping them in boiling water.

Functions: Nourishes the heart and quiets the spirit, moistens the intestines and frees the stools

Indications: This tea is suitable for the treatment of insomnia, frequent dreams, and palpitations due to blood vacuity being unable to nourish the heart. It is also for senile or postpartum blood vacuity intestinal dryness and constipation.

Jasmine Flower Tea (*Mo Li Hua Cha*)

Sweetflag rhizome, *i.e.*, Rhizoma Acori Graminei (*Shi Chang Pu*)   6 grams
Jasmine flower, *i.e.*, Flos Jasmini (*Mo Li Hua*)   6 grams
Green Tea, *i.e.*, Folium Camelliae Theae (*Qing Cha*)   10 grams

Method of administration: Grind these three herbs into a coarse powder. Soak in boiling water and drink at any time of the day. Use 1 packet per day.

Functions: Rectifies the qi, transforms dampness, and quiets the spirit

Indications: This tea is suitable for the treatment of palpitations, forgetfulness, insomnia with profuse dreams, and neurosis due to phlegm confounding the portals of the heart. In this case, there are usually elements of liver depression/qi stagnation and depressive heat. Therefore, one would also look for a reddish tongue with a slimy, yellow coating, and a wiry, slippery pulse.

Quiet the Spirit Tea (*An Shen Cha*)

Dens Draconis (*Long Chi*)   10 grams
Sweetflag rhizome, *i.e.*, Rhizoma Acori Graminei (*Shi Chang Pu*)   3 grams

Method of administration: First boil the fossilized teeth in water for 10 minutes and then add the Sweetflag and continue boiling for another 10-15 minutes. Drink this at any time, 1-2 packets per day.

Functions: Quiets the heart and calms the spirit

Indications: This tea is suitable for disquieted heart spirit, frightened heart and timorous gallbladder, and trouble sleeping.

Wind Stroke Teas

In TCM, cerebral vascular accident (CVA) or stroke is called "wind stroke." It is called this because it happens suddenly and its symptoms are variable with fast changes. The main symptoms of stroke are sudden loss of consciousness accompanied by deviation of the eyes and mouth, hemiplegia, or inhibited speech. If there is no loss of consciousness, there may be only a deviated face. Clinically, wind stroke is divided into two types: channels and network vessels stroke and viscera and bowel stroke. In the former, there is no loss of consciousness and the condition is light. In the latter, there is loss of consciousness and the condition is severe. This condition includes cerebral hemorrhage, cerebral thrombosis, cerebral embolism, subarachnoid hemorrhage, and cerebrovascular spasm as well as facial paralysis.

Burdock Root Tea (*Niu Bang Gen Cha*)

Burdock root, *i.e.*, Radix Arctii Lappae (*Niu Bang Gen*)	250 grams

Note: Burdock root is often sold in health food stores under the Japanese name of *gobo*.

Method of administration: Juice the root in a juicing machine or grind the root and press out the juice. Drink this liquid, 1 packet per day.

Functions: Dispels wind evils

Indications: This tea is suitable for the treatment of acute stroke, sudden strike by evil wind, and falling unconscious with change of facial complexion due to liver yang hyperactivity giving rise to liver wind stirring internally.

Quicken the Blood Tea (*Huo Xue Cha*)

Safflower, *i.e.*, Flos Carthami Tinctorii (*Hong Hua*)	5 grams
Sandalwood, *i.e.*, Lignum Santali Albi (*Tan Xiang*)	5 grams
Green Tea, *i.e.*, Folium Camelliae Theae (*Lu Cha*)	1 gram

Brown sugar (*Hong Tang*)   25 grams

Method of administration: Boil the above ingredients. Use 1 packet per day and drink warm at any time.

Functions: Quickens the blood and transforms stasis

Indications: This tea is suitable for the treatment of cerebral thrombosis, hypertension, angiocardiopathy, thrombus thromboangiitis obliterans (Buerger's disease), anemia, and dysmenorrhea when exhibiting a blood stasis pattern. Although strokes typically occur due to liver yang hyperactivity giving rise to internal stirring of liver wind, once the stroke occurs, the sequela are due to a varying combination of wind (tremors), phlegm obstruction (aphasia and paralysis), qi and blood vacuity (paralysis), and blood stasis (paralysis).

5
Musculoskeletal Diseases

Bi Syndrome Teas

In TCM, *bi* syndrome refers to various types of muscle, sinews, bone, and joint pain. There may also be symptoms of numbness, heaviness, inhibited flexion and extension, or swollen joints with burning heat. If pain is the dominant factor, it is called painful *bi* or cold *bi*. If the pain is migratory, it is called wind *bi* or moving *bi*. If the four limbs are numb with obvious heaviness, it is called fixed or damp *bi*. If there is palpable inflammation, redness, and swelling with painful joints that cannot flex and extend, this is called heat *bi*. Rheumatism, rheumatoid arthritis, rheumatic fever, gout, and sciatica in Western medicine all belong to this Chinese disease category.

Silkworm & Alpinia Tea (*Jiang Can Liang Jiang Cha*)

Bombyx Batryticatus (*Bai Jiang Can*)	Equal amounts
Rhizoma Alpiniae Officinari (*Gao Liang Jiang*)	Equal amounts
Green Tea, *i.e.*, Folium Camelliae Theae (*Lu Cha*)	A suitable amount

Method of administration: Grind the first two herbs into a fine powder and mix well. Store this powder in a container and seal. Use 3 grams of this powder each time, 2 times per day. Boil with 3-5 grams of green Tea. Another method is to steep the powder and green Tea in boiling water, stir well, and drink.

Functions: Scatters cold, dispels wind, and stops pain

Indications: This tea is suitable for the treatment of cold, damp *bi* pain, headache, and head wind. Individuals who have cold and painful joints of the four limbs or have *bi* pain when the weather is cloudy, rainy, cold, and damp may be helped by this formula.

Angelica Pubescens Tea (*Du Huo Cha*)

Radix Angelicae Pubescentis (*Du Huo*)   20 grams

Method of administration: Boil the herb in water. Remove the dregs and drink freely as a tea.

Functions: Dispels wind, scatters cold, and disinhibits dampness

Indications: This tea is suitable for the treatment of wind *bi* that is due to wind, cold, and/or dampness invading the joints and the channels and network vessels, thus causing pain in the joints with no fixed location.

Chinese Quince Fruit Tea (*Mu Gua Cha*)

Chinese quince fruit, *i.e.*, Fructus Chaenomelis Lagenariae
    (*Mu Gua*)   15-20 grams
Southern Cortex Radicis Acanthopanacis (*Nan Wu Jia Pi*)   12 grams
Mix-fried licorice root, *i.e.*, mix-fried Radix Glycyrrhizae
    Uralensis (*Zhi Gan Cao*)   6 grams

Method of administration: Boil the above ingredients in 500ml of water for 15 minutes and then drink the resulting liquid. These ingredients can be resoaked boiled again with water for the next dose. Use 1 packet per day. Drink this freely as a tea.

Functions: Soothes the sinews and quickens the network vessels, harmonizes the stomach and transforms dampness

Indications: This tea is suitable for the treatment of bone and joint pain due to damp, hypertonicity of the limbs, and foot qi with swelling.

Sophora & Walnut Tea (*Huai Tao Cha*)

Fructus Sophorae Japonicae (*Huai Jiao*)	15 grams
Walnut, *i.e.*, Semen Juglandis Regiae (*Hu Tao Ren*)	15 grams
Sesame seeds, *i.e.*, Semen Sesami Indici (*Zhi Ma*)	15 grams
Tea leaves, *i.e.*, Folium Camelliae Theae (*Cha Ye*)	15 grams

Method of administration: Place the above herbs in a pot, add 2 bowls of water, and boil until 1 bowl of water is left. Use 1 packet per day and drink this tea while hot.

Functions: Supplements the kidneys and strengthens the bones, dispels wind and stops pain

Indications: This tea is suitable for the treatment of rheumatoid arthritis due to a combination of kidney vacuity and wind dampness.

Epimedium & Chinese Quince Tea (*Xian Ling Mu Gua Cha*)

Herba Epimedii (*Xian Ling Pi*)	15 grams
Chinese quince fruit, *i.e.*, Fructus Chaenomelis Lagenariae (*Mu Gua*)	12 grams
Licorice root, *i.e.*, Radix Glycyrrhizae Uralensis (*Gan Cao*)	9 grams

Method of administration: Boil the above three herbs with water, remove the dregs, and drink the tea. Another method is to grind the herbs into a coarse powder and steep them in hot water in a thermos. Use 1 packet per day, drunk warm at any time.

Functions: Soothes the sinews and frees the network vessels, dispels wind and eliminates damp, disinhibits blockage and stops pain

Indications: This tea is suitable for the treatment of wind damp *bi* pain with numbness in the four limbs. It is especially useful for chronic *bi* conditions where there is an element of underlying kidney vacuity.

Job's Tears Barley & Ledebouriella Tea (*Yi Mi Fang Feng Cha*)

Job's Tears barley, *i.e.*, Semen Coicis Lachryma-jobi (*Yi Yi Ren*)   30 grams
Radix Ledebouriellae Divaricatae (*Fang Feng*)   10 grams

Method of administration: Decoct the above two herbs with water, remove the dregs, and use the liquid. Use 1 packet per day. Drink this as a tea, 1-2 doses per day. One week equals 1 course of treatment.

Functions: Dispels wind and eliminates dampness, frees the channels and diffuses *bi*

Indications: This tea is suitable for treating wind damp invading the channels and network vessels causing heaviness and pain with slightly swollen and hot limb joints. In other words, there is wind damp *bi* with an element of heat.

Strengthening the Sinews & Bones Tea (*Qiang Zhuang Jin Gu Cha*)

Herba Siegesbeckiae Orientalis (*Xi Xian Cao*)   15 grams

Method of administration: Rinse the herb, boil with water, discard the dregs, and use the liquid. Drink as a tea.

Functions: Dispels wind dampness, disinhibits the joints, and downbears (blood) pressure

Indications: This tea is suitable for the treatment of numbness of the four limbs, pain in the sinews and bones, weakness in the low back and knees, and hypertension.

Low Back & Leg Pain Teas

In TCM, low back and leg pain is usually due to contraction of cold and dampness, wind heat, traumatic injury, such as sprain and strain, physical weakness due to chronic illness, and uncontrollable sexual intemperance. In Western medicine, low back pain may be due to kidney disease, rheumatic disease, musculoskeletal over-taxation, or traumatic injury.

Cibotium Tea (*Gou Ji Cha*)

Rhizoma Cibotii Barometsis (*Gou Ji*)   20 grams

Method of administration: Boil this herb with water and drink as a tea, 1 packet per day.

Functions: Dispels cold and dampness and frees the channels and network vessels

Indications: This tea is suitable for the treatment of cold damp low back pain. This pain is due to wind, cold, and dampness stagnating the channels and network vessels. Thus the qi and blood does not move smoothly. This causes the lumbar area to feel cold, painful, and heavy. It is uncomfortable to turn the body. This pain decreases with heat and increases with cold.

Gusuibu Tea (*Gu Sui Bu Cha*)

Rhizoma Gusuibu (*Gu Sui Bu*)   50 grams
Cinnamon twig, *i.e.*, Ramulus Cinnamomi (*Gui Zhi*)   15 grams

Method of administration: Boil these two herbs together with water. Use 1 packet per day. Drink the resulting liquid as a tea.

Functions: Quickens the blood and scatters cold, supplements the kidneys and strengthens the low back

Indications: This tea is suitable for the treatment of wrenching and contusion of the low back.

Boost the Kidneys Beverage Tea (*Yi Shen Yin Zhi*)

Fructus Ligustri Lucidi (*Nu Zhen Zi*)	50 grams
Herba Ecliptae Prostratae (*Han Lian Cao*)	50 grams
Fructus Lycii Chinensis (*Gou Qi Zi*)	50 grams
Chrysanthemum flower, *i.e.*, Flos Chrysanthemi Morifolii (*Bai Ju Hua*)	30 grams
White sugar (*Bai Tang*)	Amount to taste

Method of administration: Boil the first four herbs with water, discard the dregs, and reserve the liquid. Add the white sugar while hot. Use 1 packet per day. Drink warm as a tea at any time.

Functions: Supplements the kidneys and boosts the essence

Indications: This tea is suitable for the treatment of kidney vacuity with low back pain, dizziness and tinnitus, and lower limb pain and weakness.

Acanthopanax Tea (*Wu Jia Pi Cha*)

Cortex Radicis Acanthopanacis (*Wu Jia Pi*)	15-20 grams
Mix-fried licorice root, *i.e.*, mix-fried Radix Glycyrrhizae Uralensis (*Zhi Gan Cao*)	6 grams

Method of administration: Boil these two herbs briefly. Take frequently, 1 packet per day.

Functions: Strengthens the sinews and bones, dispels wind and dampness, and stops pain

Indications: This tea is suitable for the treatment of a weak constitution with aching low back and knees, weak lower limbs, and wind damp *bi* pain.

Lateral Costal Pain Teas

Lateral costal pain means pain on one or both sides of the lateral costal region. Anger, external injury, essence blood depletion and detriment causing liver qi depression and binding, static blood blocking internally, liver yin insufficiency, or damp heat in the liver and gallbladder can all cause lateral costal pain. In Western medicine, diseases of the liver and gallbladder, intercostal neuralgia, herpes zoster, and pleurisy may all be accompanied by lateral costal pain. The following medicinal tea formulas should be selected based on a TCM pattern discrimination.

Malted Barley Tea (*Mai Ya Cha*)

Malted barley sprouts, *i.e.,* Fructus Germinatus Hordei Vulgaris (*Mai Ya*)	10 grams
Green Tea, *i.e.,* Folium Camelliae Theae (*Lu Cha*)	1 gram

Method of administration: Quickly rinse the barley sprouts with cold water, place in a small steel pot, and add ½ bowl of water. After boiling over medium heat, pour the liquid immediately into a cup with the green Tea. Cover the cup for 5 minutes and then drink. Later, one may add more boiled water to the cup and drink again and again while hot until the tea becomes weak.

Functions: Courses the liver and rectifies the qi, opens the stomach and increases the appetite, restrains lactation and disperses distention

Indications: This tea is suitable for the treatment of liver depression/qi stagnation with distention and pain in both lateral costal regions and poor appetite. It is perfect for overweight individuals.

Contraindications: Individuals with a weak constitution should be cautious when using this formula or should use it at only a half dose. It is contraindicated during pregnancy and in nursing women.

Rose Flower Tea (*Mei Gui Hua Cha*)

Flos Rosae Rugosae (*Mei Gui Hua*)   6-10 grams

Method of administration: Place the dry rose flower petals in a teapot, pour in boiling water, and cover for a moment. Drink this warm at any time.

Functions: Moves the qi and harmonizes the blood, courses the liver and resolves depression

Indications: This tea is suitable for the treatment of liver/stomach qi pain, pain in the chest and lateral costal regions with distention and fullness, pain in the epigastrium which feels better after belching, and no desire for food.

Malted Barley & Green Tangerine Peel Tea (*Mai Ya Qing Pi Cha*)

Uncooked malted barley sprouts, *i.e.*, uncooked Fructus
    Germinatus Hordei Vulgaris (*Sheng Mai Ya*)   30 grams
Immature tangerine peel, *i.e.*, Pericarpium Citri Reticulatae
    Viride (*Qing Pi*)   10 grams

Method of administration: Boil these two ingredients, discard the dregs, and reserve the liquid. Drink warm at any time.

Functions: Courses the liver, rectifies the qi, and harmonizes the stomach

Indications: This tea is suitable for the treatment of liver depression/qi stagnation, distention and pain in both lateral costal regions caused by transverse counterflow invading the stomach, and no pleasure in food.

Citron Fruit & Ginger Tea (*Fo Shou Jiang Tang Cha*)

Fructus Citri Sarcrodactylis (*Fo Shou*)   10 grams
Uncooked ginger, *i.e.*, uncooked Rhizoma Zingiberis (*Sheng Jiang*) 6 grams

White sugar (*Bai Tang*)   Amount to taste

Method of administration: Boil the citron fruit and ginger together. Discard the dregs and add the white sugar. Drink this freely any time.

Functions: Courses the liver and harmonizes the stomach

Indications: This tea is suitable for the treatment of liver/stomach disharmony causing tightness in the chest and epigastrium, lateral costal distention and pain periodic nausea and vomiting, frequent sighing, and no pleasure in eating.

Sappan Wood Tea (*Su Mu Cha*)

Lignum Sappan (*Su Mu*)   12 grams

Method of administration: Boil the sappan wood with water. Discard the dregs and drink the liquid.

Functions: Dispels stasis and frees the network vessels, quickens the blood and stops pain

Indications: This tea is suitable for the treatment of lateral costal pain due to impact injury resulting in blood stasis. In this case, there is stabbing pain in the lateral costal region and ribs. When pressed, the pain gets worse, and the painful spot is fixed in location.

Contraindications: Do not use this tea during pregnancy.

Cinnamon Twig Tea (*Gui Zhi Cha*)

Cinnamon twig, *i.e.*, Ramulus Cinnamomi (*Gui Zhi*)   30 grams
Fructus Aurantii (*Zhi Ke*)   30 grams
Uncooked ginger, *i.e.*, uncooked Rhizoma Zingiberis (*Sheng Jiang*)   2 slices

Method of administration: Boil these three ingredients with water. Discard the dregs and drink the liquid.

Functions: Scatters cold and warms the channels, quickens the blood and stops pain

Indications: This tea is suitable for the treatment of cold pain in both the lateral costal regions. This type of pain is usually due to the cold evils entering internally after injury causing cold pain in both lateral costal regions and ribs as well as a feeling of cold all over the body and an obvious fear of cold.

Contraindications: Use cautiously during pregnancy.

6
Metabolic, Neurologic & Endocrine Diseases

Diabetes Teas

Diabetes mellitus is a disease due to hypoinsulinism which causes a disturbance in carbohydrate metabolism. Its main clinical symptoms are increased blood sugar, glucose in the urine, and the "three polys": polyphagia, polydypsia, and polyuria. Diabetes is a common disease in the middle-aged and elderly. It belongs to the category of "wasting & thirst" in TCM. The occurrence of the disease is mainly related to the lungs, spleen and stomach, and kidneys. Thus, clinically, it is divided into the upper, middle, and lower three wastings and is treated by differentiating patterns associated with one or more of the three burners.

Trichosanthes Tea (*Tian Hua Fen Cha*)

Radix Trichosanthis Kirlowii (*Tian Hua Fen*)   125 grams

Method of administration: Grind the trichosanthes into a coarse powder. Use 15-20 grams each time, steeping this in boiling water. Drink this frequently throughout the day.

Functions: Clears heat, engenders fluids, and stops thirst

Indications: This tea is suitable for the treatment of thirsting and wasting characterized primarily by excessive thirst due to heat in the stomach causing damage to lung and stomach fluids. It can also be used for lung dryness cough with blood-streaked phlegm.

Contraindications: Do not take this tea during pregnancy. It may cause a miscarriage.

Nourishing the Stomach Tea (*Yang Wei Cha*)

Radix Glehniae Littoralis (*Bei Sha Shen*)	15 grams
Tuber Ophiopogonis Japonici (*Mai Men Dong*)	15 grams
Uncooked Radix Rehmanniae (*Sheng Di*)	15 grams
Solomon's seal, *i.e.*, Rhizoma Polygonati Odorati (*Yu Zhu*)	5 grams

Method of administration: Grind the above herbs into a coarse powder, boil with water, and use the liquid. Drink this as a tea, using 1 packet per day.

Functions: Boosts the stomach and engenders fluids

Indications: This tea is suitable for the treatment of upper wasting disease, heat disease damaging yin, and vexatious thirst disease.

Ginger & Salt Tea (*Jiang Yan Cha*)

Uncooked ginger, *i.e.*, uncooked Rhizoma Zingiberis (*Sheng Jiang*)	2 slices
Salt (*Yan*)	4.5 grams
Green Tea, *i.e.*, Folium Camelliae Theae (*Lu Cha*)	6 grams

Method of administration: Boil the three ingredients with water. Drink the resulting tea freely at any time. Use 1-2 packets per day.

Functions: Clears heat and moistens dryness, engenders fluids and stops thirst

Indications: This tea is suitable for the treatment of thirst, excessive drinking, vexatious heat in the heart, and copious urine.

Umeboshi Tea (*Wu Mei Cha*)

Umeboshi, *i.e.*, Fructus Pruni Mume (*Wu Mei*)	50 grams

Method of administration: Boil the umeboshi with water or soak in boiling water for 10 minutes. Use 1 packet per day. Drink this warm as a tea at any time.

Functions: Engenders fluids and stops thirst

Indications: This tea is suitable for the treatment of diabetes wasting and thirst disease due to stomach yin vacuity. Interestingly, there may also be the complication of damp heat in the lower burner affecting either the bladder or large intestine.

Melon Peel Tea (*Gua Pi Cha*)

Chinese wax gourd peel, *i.e.*, Exocarpium Benincasae Hispidae (*Dong Gua Pi*)	10 grams
Watermelon peel, *i.e.*, Exocarpium Citrulli Vulgaris (*Xi Gua Pi*)	10 grams
Radix Trichosanthis Kirlowii (*Tian Hua Fen*)	8 grams

Method of administration: Wash these three ingredients separately and chop them into small slices. Place in a pot, add water, and boil for 10-15 minutes. Use 1 packet per day. Drink the liquid as a tea.

Functions: Clears heat, engenders fluid, and stops thirst

Indications: This tea is suitable for the treatment of diabetic patients with thirst, summerheat vexatious thirst, and inhibited urination.

Dioscorea Tea (*Shan Yao Cha*)

Radix Dioscoreae Oppositae (*Shan Yao*)	250 grams

Method of administration: Boil this herb with water and then filter the liquid. Use 1 packet per day. Drink this freely as a tea.

Functions: Supplements the qi, nourishes yin, and stops thirst

111

Indications: This tea is suitable for the treatment of diabetic patients with a spleen/kidney vacuity and an element of yin vacuity as well.

Simple Obesity Teas

If a person's weight is 20% above normal, this is called simple obesity. Not only does obesity affect an individual's general physical abilities, but it can also be a contributing and complicating factor in many diseases. Thus, it is important to adopt active and vigorous measures for the prevention and treatment of obesity.

Lose Weight Tea (*Jian Fei Cha*)

Folium Nelumbinis Nuciferae (*He Ye*)	60 grams
Uncooked hawthorn fruit, *i.e.*, uncooked Fructus Crataegi (*Sheng Shan Zha*)	10 grams
Job's Tears barley, *i.e.*, Semen Coicis Lachryma-jobi (*Yi Yi Ren*)	10 grams
Tangerine peel, *i.e.*, Pericarpium Citri Reticulatae (*Ju Pi*)	5 grams

Method of administration: Grind all of the above ingredients into a fine powder and mix evenly. Place this powder in a thermos and soak in boiling water. Use 1 packet per day, drinking it at any time. Take this tea continuously for 100 days.

Functions: Rectifies the qi and moves water, lowers fat and transforms turbidity

Indications: This tea is suitable for the treatment of simple obesity and high cholesterol. It also benefits coronary heart disease and hypertension.

Sweet Milk Tea (*Tian Nai Cha*)

Milk (*Niu Nai*)	100ml
Tea leaves, *i.e.*, Folium Camelliae Theae (*Cha Ye*)	8 grams

White sugar (*Bai Tang*)   Amount to taste

Method of administration: Place the Tea leaves into a cup and soak in boiling water. Place the milk into a pot and boil. Add the white sugar, and then add in the Tea water.

Functions: Supplements vacuity and boosts the stomach, engenders fluids and lubricates the intestines.

Indications: This tea is suitable for the treatment of obesity with lassitude of the spirit, indigestion, and constipation.

Lotus & Hawthorn Tea (*He Zha Cha*)

Fresh Folium Nelumbinis Nuciferae (*Xian He Ye*)	65 grams
Hawthorn fruit, *i.e.*, Fructus Crataegi (*Shan Zha*)	15 grams
Job's Tears barley, *i.e.*, Semen Coicis Lachryma-jobi (*Yi Yi Ren*)	15 grams
Tangerine peel, i.e., Pericarpium Citri Reticulatae (*Ju Pi*)	7 grams
Semen Cassiae Torae (*Jue Ming Zi*)	15 grams
Rhizoma Alismatis (*Ze Xie*)	12 grams

Method of administration: Dry the lotus leaf first. Then grind all the ingredients together into a powder. Place this powder into a thermos and steep in boiling water. Use 1 packet per day and take continuously for 30 days.

Functions: Rectifies the qi and percolates dampness

Indications: This tea is suitable for the treatment of simple obesity and high cholesterol due to spleen vacuity and dampness with an element of liver depression or hyperactivity.

Lotus Leaf Tea (*He Ye Cha*)

Folium Nelumbinis Nuciferae (*He Ye*)	10 grams
Green Tea, *i.e.*, Folium Camelliae Theae (*Lu Cha*)	10 grams

113

Method of administration: Soak these two ingredients in boiled water. Drink this whenever thirsty.

Functions: Clears heat and cools the blood, fortifies the spleen and disinhibits water

Indications: This tea is suitable for the treatment of obesity and high cholesterol.

Wu Long Tea (*Wu Long Cha*)

Wu Long Tea, *i.e.*, Wu Long Folium Camelliae Theae (*Wu Long Cha*) 3 grams
Fructus Sophorae Japonicae (*Huai Jiao*) 18 grams
Radix Polygoni Multiflori (*He Shou Wu*) 30 grams
Chinese wax gourd peel, *i.e.*, Exocarpium Benincasae Hispidae
    (*Dong Gua Pi*) 18 grams
Hawthorn fruit (without the core), *i.e.*, Fructus Crataegi
    (*Shan Zha Rou*) 15 grams

Note: Wu Long Tea is a specific type of Tea which is said to supplement the kidneys.

Method of administration: Boil the last four herbs with water for 20 minutes. Use the hot liquid to steep the Wu Long Tea. Use 1 packet per day, drunk at any time.

Functions: Disperses and decreases lipids, fortifies the body, and boosts longevity

Indications: This tea is suitable for the treatment of obesity and hyperlipidemia associated with liver/kidney yin vacuity and hyperactivity of liver yang.

Pu Er Tea (*Pu Er Cha*)

Pu Er Tea, *i.e.*, Folium Camelliae Theae (*Pu Er Cha*)   6 grams

Note: Pu Er Tea is believed to be especially beneficial to the digestion.

Method of administration: Soak the Tea in a cup with boiling water for 10 minutes or decoct with water for 5 minutes. Use 1 packet per day. Drink this warm at any time.

Functions: Fortifies the spleen, disperses food, and reduces fat

Indications: This tea is suitable for the treatment of obesity, nausea and vomiting, cough with copious phlegm, and acute diseases such as cholera and sunstroke.

Artemisia Capillaris Fat Reducing Tea (*Yin Chen Jian Fei Cha*)

Herba Artemisiae Capillaris (*Yin Chen Hao*)	Equal amount
Fructus Rosae Laevigatae (*Jin Ying Zi*)	Equal amount
Semen Cassiae Torae (*Jue Ming Zi*)	Equal amount
Hawthorn fruit, *i.e.*, Fructus Crataegi (*Shan Zha*)	Equal amount
Folium Nelumbinis Nuciferae (*He Ye*)	Equal amount

Method of administration: Dry these herbs and grind each into a coarse powder, screening it 14-20 times. Mix the coarse powders together and place them in a container. Seal the container for storage. Use 3-6 grams of powder one time per day, soaking it in boiling water for 5 minutes. One may also put this powder into filter paper to make tea bags.

Functions: Courses the liver and rectifies the qi, clears heat and disinhibits dampness, reduces fat

Indications: This tea is suitable for the treatment of obesity due to liver depression affecting the spleen.

Mulberry Twig Tea (*Sang Zhi Cha*)

Tender, *i.e.,* fresh mulberry twigs, *i.e.*, Ramulus Mori Albi
   (*Nen Sang Zhi*)   20 grams

Method of administration: Chop the mulberry twigs into thin slices, place in a teacup, and steep in boiling water for 10 minutes. Use 1 packet per day. Drink this as a tea at any time. Take continuously for 2-3 months.

Functions: Dispels wind dampness and moves water and qi

Indications: This tea is suitable for the treatment of obesity and joint pain.

High Cholesterol Teas

High cholesterol or hyperlipidemia has to do with the abnormal metabolism of lipids. Clinically, it refers to higher than normal levels of blood lipids. This may or may not be accompanied by symptoms of dizziness, palpitations, numbness in the limbs, and feelings of oppression in the chest. In TCM, this condition is similar to "phlegm turbidity" and certain of its symptoms fall under the categories of "palpitations," "dizziness," and "chest oppression." In treatment, the main focus is on regulating the functions of the viscera and bowels.

Hawthorn & Lotus Leaf Tea (*Shan Zha He Ye Cha*)

Hawthorn fruit, *i.e.*, Fructus Crataegi (*Shan Zha*)   15 grams
Folium Nelumbinis Nuciferae (*He Ye*)   12 grams

Method of administration: Chop these two ingredients into fine pieces and boil with water. The herbs may also be steeped in boiling water. In either case, drink the heavy liquid. Use 1 packet per day. Drink this freely as a tea at any time.

Functions: Disperses lipids and transforms stagnation, lowers pressure, and reduces fat

Indications: This tea is suitable for the treatment of hypertension, high cholesterol, and obesity.

Dispersing Stagnation & Reducing Fat Tea (*Xiao Zhi Jian Fei Cha*)

Green Tea, *i.e.*, Folium Camellia Theae (*Lu Cha*)	6 grams
Rhubarb root, *i.e.*, Radix Et Rhizoma Rhei (*Da Huang*)	2 grams

Method of administration: Soak these two ingredients in boiling water. Use 1 packet per day and drink freely as a tea.

Functions: Clears heat and drains fire, frees the stool disperses accumulation, reduces fat

Indications: This tea is suitable for the treatment of high cholesterol and obesity when associated with a *tai yang* constitutional body type with liver depression and/or hyperactivity and chronic constipation. Frequent drinking of this tea can delay debilitation due to aging.

Contraindications: Rhubarb is a purgative and should be used with caution in pregnancy and postpartum.

Fortify the Body & Reduce Lipids Tea (*Jian Shen Jiang Zhi Cha*)

Green Tea, *i.e.*, Folium Camelliae Theae (*Lu Cha*)	10 grams
Radix Polygoni Multiflori (*He Shou Wu*)	10 grams
Rhizoma Alismatis (*Ze Xie*)	10 grams
Radix Salviae Miltiorrhizae (*Dan Shen*)	10 grams

Method of administration: Boil these ingredients in water and use the liquid. Use 1 packet per day.

Functions: Quickens the blood and disinhibits dampness, lowers lipids and reduces fat

Indications: This tea is suitable for the treatment of hyperlipidemia and obesity associated with blood stasis.

Hawthorn Fruit Lipid Reducing Tea (*Shan Zha Jiang Zhi Cha*)

Fresh hawthorn fruit, *i.e.*, fresh Fructus Crataegi (*Xian Shan Zha*	30 grams
Uncooked Flos Immaturus Sophorae Japonicae	
(*Sheng Huai Hua Mi*)	5 grams
Tender Folium Nelumbinis Nuciferae (*Nen He Ye*)	15 grams
Semen Cassiae Torae (*Jue Ming Zi*)	10 grams
White sugar (*Bai Tang*)	Amount to taste

Method of administration: Boil the four herbs. When the hawthorn fruit is well cooked, crush it with a soup spoon, and cook for another 10 minutes. Strain the liquid and add white sugar while still hot. Drink this warm or cool at any time. Take 1 packet per day.

Functions: Transforms stasis and moves stagnation

Indications: This tea is suitable for the treatment of high cholesterol exhibiting a blood stasis pattern.

Thyroid Enlargement Teas

Enlargement of the thyroid may be due to poor iodine assimilation, shortage of iodine in the diet, tumors, thyroiditis, inflammation from infection, or hyperfunction or hypofunction of the thyroid. In TCM, enlargement of the thyroid belongs to the category of "goiter."

Kelp Tea (*Kun Bu Cha*)

Kelp, *i.e.*, Thallus Algae (*Kun Bu*)	500 grams

Method of administration: Soak the dry kelp in cold water for 24 hours. Then cut into fine threads. Stir-fry dry in an iron pot. Use 3 grams of the kelp each time by soaking it in boiled water and drinking the liquid slowly. Take once per day.

Functions: Clears heat and transforms phlegm, softens the hard and scatters nodulation

Indications: This tea is mainly for simple thyroid enlargement, the prevention of thyroid dysfunction, and the treatment of hypertension and arteriosclerosis associated with phlegm obstruction.

Leechee & Apricot Kernel Tea (*Li Zhi Xing Ren Cha*)

Dried leechee fruit, *i.e.*, dried Fructus Litchi Chinensis (*Gan Li Zhi*)   50 grams
Apricot kernel, *i.e.*, Semen Pruni Armeniacae (*Xing Ren*)   10 grams
Tea leaves, *i.e.*, Folium Camelliae Theae (*Cha Ye*)   3 grams
White sugar (*Bai Tang*)   Amount to taste

Method of administration: Place the first three ingredients in a pot, add water, and boil for 20 minutes. Discard the dregs, saving the liquid, and add the white sugar and stir evenly. Use 1 packet per day. Drink this freely as a tea.

Functions: Rectifies the qi and transforms phlegm in order to clear phlegm nodulation

Indications: This tea is suitable for the treatment of thyroid enlargement and thyroid tumors due to liver depression with phlegm nodulation.

Sargassium & Cassia Seed Tea (*Hai Ming Cha*)

Herba Sargassii (*Hai Zao*)   30 grams
Semen Cassiae Torae (*Jue Ming Zi*)   25 grams

119

Method of administration: Wash these two ingredients well and place in a pot. Then add water. Boil for 20 minutes and use the liquid. Use 1 packet per day and drink it slowly as a tea.

Functions: Clears, cools, and discharges heat, transforms phlegm and scatters nodulation, clears heat and disinhibits water

Indications: This tea is suitable for the treatment of thyroid enlargement, water swelling, chronic tracheitis, cough, hypertension, and laryngitis due to phlegm nodulation and liver depression with upward counterflow and depressive heat.

Insomnia Teas

Insomnia refers to the inability to sleep or to sleep which is interrupted by wakefulness. There are different types of insomnia, such as difficulty in falling asleep, awaking easily after falling asleep, inability to return to sleep again after waking, and the inability to sleep throughout the entire night. There may be accompanying symptoms of dizziness, headache, heart palpitations, and impaired memory. In TCM, there are various reasons for insomnia. For instance, qi depression may transform into fire which then harasses and stirs the heart spirit. It may also be due to stomach disharmony and the phlegm heat harassing internally or to yin vacuity with fire effulgence. If the qi of the heart and gallbladder are vacuous, the spirit is shaken and easily frightened. All of these can influence the heart spirit and cause insomnia. Clinically, treatment is usually divided into two patterns—vacuity and repletion. The vacuity pattern focuses on enriching yin, nourishing the heart, fortifying the spleen, and quieting the spirit, while the repletion pattern focuses on coursing the liver, draining heat, and transforming phlegm.

Mulberry Tea (*Sang Shen Cha*)

Mulberry fruit, *i.e.*, Fructus Mori Albi (*Sang Shen*)   15 grams

Method of administration: Boil the mulberries in water. Remove the dregs and reserve the liquid. Use 1 packet per day.

Functions: Enriches and supplements kidney yin, clears the heart and drains the fire

Indications: This tea is suitable for the treatment of a weak constitution after illness with loss of interaction between the heart and kidneys causing insomnia, dream emission or unconscious loss of seminal fluid during dreaming, heart palpitations, and impaired memory.

Juncus & Lophatherum Tea (*Deng Xin Zhu Ye Cha*)

Medulla Junci Effusi (*Deng Xin Cao*)   60 grams
Fresh Herba Lophatheri Gracilis (*Xian Dan Zhu Ye*)   60 grams

Method of administration: Boil these two ingredients in water. Drink the resulting tea warm at any time, 1 packet per day.

Functions: Quiets the spirit and stabilizes the will, settles fright and clears the heart

Indications: This tea is suitable for treating insomnia, easily becoming frightened and angry, heart palpitations, and impaired memory due to heart fire.

Lophatherum Quiet the Heart Tea (*Zhu Ye Ning Xin Cha*)

Fresh Herba Lophatheri Gracilis (*Xian Dan Zhu Ye*)   60 grams

Method of administration: Place the herb in a pot, add water, and make into a strong tea. Use 1 packet per day, taken in 2 divided doses, 1 in the morning and 1 in the afternoon.

Functions: Clears heat and eliminates vexation, stops thirst and quiets the heart

Indications: This tea is suitable for the treatment of heart vexation, thirst, and troubled sleep after a heat disease where there is still heat lingering in and harassing the heart.

Quiet Sleep Tea (*An Shui Cha*)

Medulla Junci Effusi (*Deng Xin Cao*)   10-20 grams

Method of administration: Boil the herb with water. Use 1 packet per day. Drink warm at any time.

Functions: Calms the heart and quiets the spirit, clears the heart and eliminates vexation

Indications: This tea is suitable for the treatment of insomnia and vexation of the heart as well as infant night crying with vexation of the heart due to heat in the heart.

Sour Jujube Seed Tea (*Suan Zao Ren Cha*)

Semen Ziziphi Spinosae (*Suan Zao Ren*)   9 grams
White sugar (*Bai Tang*)   Amount to taste

Method of administration: Pound the zizyphus spinosa seed into pieces. Place these pieces in a cup, pour boiling water into the cup, and allow to steep. Add white sugar for flavor.

Functions: Nourishes the heart and quiets the spirit

Indications: This tea is suitable for the treatment of vacuity vexation insomnia, heart palpitations, and racing of the heart due to heart blood and yin vacuity.

Albizzia Flower Tea (*He Huan Hua Cha*)

Mimosa tree flower, *i.e.*, Flos Albizziae Julibrissinis (*He Huan Hua*)   6 grams
White sugar (*Bai Tang*)   Amount to taste

Method of administration: Wash the mimosa tree flower well, place in a cup, and soak in boiling water. Add white sugar to taste and drink. Take 1 packet per day.

Functions: Nourishes the heart and fortifies the spleen, resolves depression and rectifies the qi

Indications: This tea is suitable for the treatment of neurasthenia, chest oppression and discomfort, and eye disease. Taken often, this formula engenders a cheerful spirit and a clear mind.

Black Bean & Wheat Tea (*Dou Mai Cha*)

Black soybeans, *i.e.*, black Semen Glycinis (*Hei Dou*)   30 grams
Blighted wheat, *i.e.*, Semen Levis Tritici Aestivi (*Fu Xiao Mai*)   30 grams
Lotus seeds, *i.e.*, Semen Nelumbinis Nuciferae (*Lian Zi*)   7 pieces
Red dates, *i.e.*, Fructus Ziziphus Jujube (*Da Zao*)   7 pieces
Crystal sugar (*Bing Tang*)   Amount to taste

Method of administration: Boil the above four herbs with water. Discard the dregs and save the liquid. Add the crystal sugar and drink when the sugar has melted.

Functions: Promotes the interaction between the heart and the kidneys

Indications: This tea is suitable for vacuity vexation insomnia, restless sleep, lassitude of the spirit, lack of strength, and impaired memory especially due to noninteraction between the heart and kidneys.

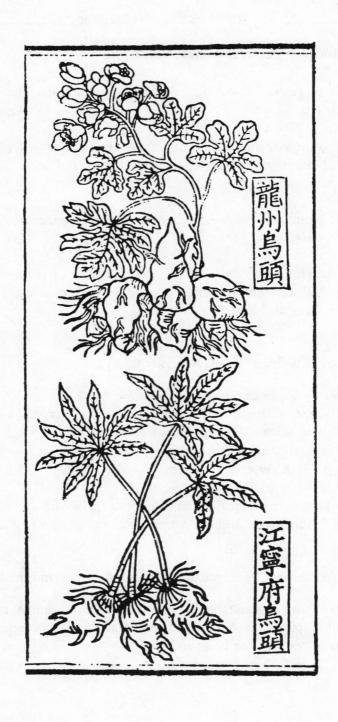

龍州烏頭

江寧府烏頭

7
Parasitic & Infectious Diseases

Worm Teas

Worms refers to parasitic diseases such as those caused by roundworms, tapeworms, pinworms, hookworms, and trichomonads that may parasitize the human intestinal tract. These parasites can affect any age group. However, roundworms and pinworms usually affect children; hookworms usually affect adults; trichomonads are usually more common in women; and the incidence of tapeworms in China depends on the region. These herbal teas get good results in expelling worms.

Expel Worms Pill Tea (*Qu Chong Wan Cha*)

Tea leaves, *i.e.*, Folium Camelliae Theae (*Cha Ye*)	9 grams
Fructificatio Polypori Mylittae (*Lei Wan*)	9 grams
Rhizoma Sparganii (*San Leng*)	9 grams
White sugar (*Bai Tang*)	10 grams
Salt (*Yan*)	3 grams

Method of administration: Grind the first three ingredients into a powder and mix well. Boil salt and white sugar, mix with the powder, and make into pills. Take 3 grams of these pills 1 time each day and then drink boiled water. Take after dinner.

Functions: Disperses stagnation, scatters nodulation, and kills worms

Indications: This tea is suitable for the treatment of roundworms and tapeworms.

Torreya Tea (*Fei Zi Cha*)

Semen Torreyae Grandis (*Fei Zi*)   30 grams

Method of administration: Stir-fry the torreya nut until it has a pleasant smell. Use 30 grams each day by steeping it in boiling water and drinking it frequently as a tea. Take it for 5-7 days continuously.

Functions: Kills worms, disperses accumulation, and moistens dryness

Indications: This tea is suitable for treating hookworms and pinworms.

Pumpkin Seed Tea (*Nan Gua Zi Cha*)

Pumpkin seeds, *i.e.,* Semen Cucurbitae Moschatae (*Nan Gua Zi*) 60 grams

Method of administration: Pound the seeds into pieces and boil these with water. Use 1 packet per day. Drink this freely as a tea at any time.

Functions: Expels worms

Indications: This tea is suitable for the treatment of tapeworms and roundworms.

White Tree Ear Tea (*Bai Mu Er Cha*)

White wood ear, *i.e.,* Fructificatio Tremellae Fuciformis
    (*Bai Mu Er*)   100 grams
White sugar (*Bai Tang*)   200 grams

Method of administration: Steep the herb in boiling water and then add the white sugar. Once a day, use 20 grams each time and drink the liquid as a tea.

Functions: Kills worms

Indications: This tea is suitable for the treatment of pinworms.

Lindera & Betel Nut Tea (*Wu Yao Bing Lang Cha*)

Betel nut, *i.e.*, Semen Arecae Catechu (*Bing Lang*)	1 piece
Radix Linderae Strychnifoliae (*Wu Yao*)	9 grams

Method of administration: Place the two herbs together in water and crush into a thick liquid. Drink this liquid with warm water.

Functions: Kills worms and settles pain

Indications: This tea is suitable for the treatment of worm accumulation abdominal pain, intolerable abdominal pain, the pain increasing with movement, and the sensation of a swollen lump sliding up and down in the abdomen.

Szechuan Pepper & Umeboshi Tea (*Hua Jiao Wu Mei Cha*)

Szechuan pepper, *i.e.*, Fructus Zanthoxyli Bungeani (*Hua Jiao*)	50 grains
Umeboshi, *i.e.*, Fructus Pruni Mume (*Wu Mei*)	10 grams

Method of administration: Pound the pepper into pieces. Then soak these pieces and the umeboshi in boiling water. Take this as a tea.

Functions: Warms the middle, quiets roundworms, and stops pain

Indications: This tea is suitable for the treatment of roundworm abdominal pain and biliary ascariasis.

Heat, *i.e.*, Febrile, Disease Teas

In Chinese medicine, heat disease generally refers to all conditions where there is fever caused by an external pathogenic contraction. The clinical symptoms are a sudden onset of illness with signs of exuberant heat, fever with no aversion to cold, rapid transmutation, and an easy tendency to transform into dryness and to damage yin. During the course of a heat disease, it is common to have symptoms of vexation and thirst or, afterwards, there may be damage to the fluids due to heat exuberance. Clinically, different herbal teas should be selected according to the different symptoms in order to either primarily clear heat and eliminate vexation or enrich yin and engender liquids.

Lotus Tea (*Ou Cha*)

Fresh lotus root, *i.e.*, Rhizoma Nelumbinis Nuciferae (*Sheng Ou*)	60 grams
White sugar (*Bai Tang*)	15 grams

Method of administration: Rinse the herb well and cut into thin slices. Place these in a pot and cook slowly with 650mls of water. After 10 minutes, add the white sugar and stir well. Use 1 packet per day. Drink as a tea.

Functions: Cools the blood, clears heat, and transforms phlegm

Indications: This tea is suitable for heat disease with vexation, thirst, red eyes, nosebleed, postpartum blood stasis, and painful voidings of hot urine. It can also resolve alcohol toxins, clear heat, and resolve summerheat.

Clear the Lungs & Allay Thirst Cooling Tea (*Qing Fei Zhi Ke Liang Cha*)

Herba Lophtheri Gracilis (*Dan Zhu Ye*)	25 grams
Fresh loquat leaf, *i.e.*, Folium Eriobotryae Japonicae (*Xian Pi Pa Ye*)	25 grams
Rhizoma Phragmitis Communis (*Lu Gen*)	25 grams
White sugar (*Bai Tang*)	Amount to taste
Table salt (*Shi Yan*)	Small amount

128

Method of administration: Rinse the first three ingredients well, chop into pieces, and place into a pot. Add 1,500ml of water and boil for 10 minutes. Discard the dregs and save the liquid. Add the salt and sugar while still hot. Use 1 packet per day, drinking it after it has cooled.

Functions: Clears heat, engenders liquids, and disinhibits urination

Indications: This tea is suitable for the treatment of vexatious thirst, summerheat, and short voidings of reddish urine. This formula can clear the lungs and stop thirst. It is a common, cooling, summertime drink.

Preventing Epidemics Teas

Pestilence refers to very contagious, wide-spread epidemics that progress quickly and are associated with severe illness. This includes Western medical epidemic infections, such as cerebrospinal meningitis and encephalitis B. The death rate of this type of infection is very high in China. However, due to the constant development of modern medicine and sanitation in China, their occurrence and death rates are decreasing on a large scale. Chinese medicinal teas can greatly contribute to the prevention of these epidemic, pestilential, and contagious diseases. The following formulas are common ones that may be chosen during epidemic seasons.

Daqingye Tea (*Da Qing Ye Cha*)

Folium Daqingye (*Da Qing Ye*)   30 grams

Method of administration: Grind the herb into a coarse powder and boil in water. Discard the dregs and drink the liquid. Use 1 packet per day. Take frequently for 3-5 days.

Functions: Clears heat, resolves toxins, and cools the blood

Indications: This tea is suitable for preventing epidemic cerebrospinal meningitis and encephalitis B.

Isatis Tea (*Ban Lan Gen Cha*)

Radix Isatidis Seu Baphicacanthi (*Ban Lan Gen*)	50 grams
Folium Daqingye (*Da Qing Ye*)	50 grams
Wild chrysanthum flower, *i.e.*, Flos Chrysanthemi Indici (*Ye Ju Hua*)	30 grams
Honeysuckle flower, *i.e.*, Flos Lonicerae Japonicae (*Jin Yin Hua*)	30 grams

Method of administration: Place the above four ingredients in a large cup and steep in boiling water. Use 1 packet per day. Drink this tea often.

Functions: Clears heat and resolves toxins

Indications: This tea is suitable for the prevention of flu and epidemic encephalitis B, epidemic hepatitis, and epidemic respiratory tract infections.

Guanzhong & Isatis Tea (*Guan Zhong Ban Lan Gen Cha*)

Rhizoma Guanzhong (*Guan Zhong*)	24 grams
Radix Isatidis Seu Baphicacanthi (*Ban Lan Gen*)	15 grams

Method of administration: Grind the above two herbs into a coarse powder and boil with water. Discard the dregs and use the liquid. Use 1 packet per day. Drink this for 3-5 days.

Functions: Clears heat and resolves toxins

Indications: This tea is suitable for the prevention of epidemic cerebrospinal meningitis.

Honeysuckle & Licorice Tea (*Yin Hua Gan Cao Cha*)

Honeysuckle flower, *i.e.*, Flos Lonicerae Japonicae (*Jin Yin Hua*)	30 grams
Licorice root, *i.e.*, Radix Glycyrrhizae Uralensis (*Gan Cao*)	3 grams

Method of administration: Grind the licorice root into a coarse powder and place in a teacup with the honeysuckle flowers. Steep these in boiling water. Use 1 packet per day. Drink freely as a tea.

Functions: Clears heat and resolves toxins

Indications: This tea is suitable for the prevention of epidemic encephalitis B and epidemic cerebrospinal meningitis.

Lymphadenopathy Tea

Lymphadenopathy belongs to the category of scrofula in TCM. It refers to pathological enlargement and hardening of the lymph nodes. These typically occur in the neck and subaxillary regions but may also be found in the inguinal region in some cases. Swollen lymph nodes may be due to chronic infection, immune deficiency, or serious disease, such as lymphoma. In TCM, swollen lymph nodes are considered to be due to liver qi depression and binding with phlegm damp congelation and gathering. This combination of depressed qi and phlegm then binds into nodulations.

Selfheal Tea (*Xia Ku Cao Cha*)

Selfheal spike, *i.e.*, Spica Prunellae Vulgaris (*Xia Ku Cao*)	30 grams
Honeysuckle flower, *i.e.*, Flos Lonicerae Japonicae (*Jin Yin Hua*)	30 grams
Herba Violae Yedoensitis Cum Radice (*Zi Hua Di Ding*)	30 grams
Crystal sugar (*Bing Tang*)	Amount to taste

Method of administration: Grind these herbs into a coarse powder, boil with water, and then use the liquid. Add the crystal sugar into the liquid and let it dissolve. Drink this frequently as a tea, 1 packet per day.

Functions: Clears heat, resolves toxins, resolves depression and scatters nodulations

Indications: This tea is suitable for the treatment of lymphadenopathy with depressive heat and phlegm nodulation.

厚朴味苦溫大溫無毒主中風傷寒頭痛寒熱驚悸。

8
External & Dermatological Diseases

Sores & Boils Teas

Sores and boils are common suppurative inflammations of the skin. They often occur in the areas of the head, armpit, or hips. Symptoms include redness, swelling, heat, and pain. Generally, these skin conditions are due to poor hygiene, infection from scratching or sweating, and infections of hair follicles or sebaceous glands.

Honeysuckle & Mung Bean Tea (*Yin Hua Lu Dou Cha*)

Honeysuckle flower, *i.e.*, Flos Lonicerae Japonicae (*Jin Yin Hua*)   30 grams
Licorice root, *i.e.,* Radix Glycyrrhizae Uralensis (*Gan Cao*)   3 grams
Mung bean, *i.e.*, Semen Phaseoli Munginis (*Lu Dou*)   15 grams

Method of administration: Boil all of these ingredients in water. Use the liquid and drink this freely as a tea.

Functions: Clears heat, resolves toxins, and disperses swelling

Indications: This tea is suitable for the prevention and treatment of summer-time boils.

Dandelion Tea (*Pu Gong Ying Cha*)

Fresh dandelion, *i.e.*, fresh Herba Taraxaci Mongolici Cum Radice
   (*Xian Pu Gong Ying*)   30 grams

Note: If using dry dandelion, use only 20 grams.

Method of administration: Wash the herb well and then boil with water. Drink the liquid as a tea. Use 1 packet per day and drink it at any time.

Functions: Clears heat and resolves toxins, disperses swelling and dissipates *yong* (carbuncles)

Indications: This tea is suitable for the treatment of summer boils and clove sore toxins.

Purslane Tea (*Ma Chi Xian Cha*)

Fresh purslane, *i.e.*, fresh Herba Portulacae Oleraceae
  (*Xian Ma Chi Xian*)   30 grams

Note: If dry, use 20 grams.

Method of administration: Rinse the herb well and boil with water. Drink the liquid as a tea. Use 1 packet per day, taken at any time.

Functions: Clears heat and resolves toxins, dispels stasis and disperses swelling

Indications: This tea is suitable for the treatment of clove sores, boils, sores, *yong* swellings, and cinnabar toxin sores, *i.e.*, erysipelas.

Urticaria Teas

Urticaria, more commonly called hives and also called nettle rash, is a vascular reaction of the skin that may be due to irritants such as physical agents, food, insect bites, medications, and pollens, or to neurogenic factors. It is characterized by transient wheels that are pale or bright red in color which occur suddenly and are usually accompanied by severe itching. In some cases, these may occur repeatedly and linger to become chronic, in some cases, lasting years and years. In TCM, hives are believed to be due to wind, dampness, and heat affecting the skin or heat that collects in the stomach with wind attacking. In chronic cases, there may also be elements of qi and/or blood, yin and/or yang vacuity.

Chinese Wax Gourd Peel Tea (*Dong Gua Pi Cha*)

Chinese wax gourd peel, *i.e.*, Exocarpium Benincasae Hispidae
    (*Dong Gua Pi*)   Any amount

Method of administration: Boil this herb with water, filter the dregs, and use the liquid. Drink this frequently as a tea.

Functions: Disinhibits water and disperses swelling

Indications: This tea is suitable for the treatment of nettle rash affecting large areas with pronounced localized edematous swelling due to accumulation of dampness.

Ginger & Vinegar Beverage Tea (*Jiang Cu Yin Cha*)

Uncooked ginger, *i.e.*, uncooked Rhizoma Zingiberis (*Sheng Jiang*)   50 grams
Brown sugar (*Hong Tang*)   100 grams
Vinegar (*Cu*)   100 grams

Method of administration: Chop the ginger into thin slices and boil with the vinegar, sugar, and water. Discard the dregs. Drink 1 small cup each time with warm water. Take 3 doses per day.

Functions: Fortifies the spleen and stomach and removes allergy

Indications: This tea is suitable for the treatment of food allergy urticaria.

Anti-allergy Tea (*Kang Min Cha*)

Umeboshi, *i.e.*, Fructus Pruni Mume (*Wu Mei*)	9 grams
Radix Ledebouriellae Divaricatae (*Fang Feng*)	9 grams
Radix Bupleuri (*Chai Hu*)	9 grams
Fructus Schisandrae Chinensis (*Wu Wei Zi*)	6 grams
Uncooked licorice root, *i.e.*, uncooked Radix Glycyrrhizae Uralensis (*Sheng Gan Cao*)	10 grams

Method of administration: Boil the above five herbs, remove the dregs, and reserve the liquid. Take 1 packet per day, drunk in 2 doses.

Functions: Clears heat and dispels dampness, dissipates wind and stops itching

Indications: This tea is suitable for the treatment of wind damp lumps due to wind heat brewing and binding as well as spleen damp wind poison with a sharp itch all over the body, fear of cold, signs of some heat, and joint pain. It also treats allergic skin rashes such as nettle rash.

Neurodermatitis Tea

Neurodermatitis is a cutaneous inflammation with itching that is often due to emotional disturbances. It often occurs symmetrically in the areas of the neck, elbows, popliteal fossa, and sacrum where the skin comes in contact with the edges of the clothes. The itch may be intense and, after scratching chronically, the skin may become lichenified or thickened. Emotional disturbances and depression typically exacerbate this condition. This condition often chronically reoccurs and lingers and is difficult to cure. In TCM, it is called oxhide *xian*.

Mugwort & Ginger Tea (*Ai Ye Lao Jiang Cha*)

Old Tea leaves, *i.e.*, old Folium Camelliae Theae (*Lao Cha Ye*)	6 grams
Mugwort leaf, *i.e.*, Folium Artemisiae Argyii (*Ai Ye*)	6 grams
Uncooked ginger, *i.e.*, uncooked Rhizoma Zingiberis Officinalis (*Sheng Jiang*)	50 grams

Purple-skin garlic, *i.e.*, purple-skinned Bulbus Allii Sativi
   (*Zi Pi Suan Tou*)   2 heads
Salt (*Yan*)   Small amount

Method of administration: Boil the first four ingredients and then add the salt. Use 1 packet every 2 days to wash the skin lesions externally.

Functions: Disperses inflammation and kills germs

Indications: This tea is suitable for the treatment of neurodermatitis.

Insect Bite Teas

Whenever a human is bitten or stung by an insect, a pathological reaction may occur to either the whole body or only locally. This is called "insect bite damage" or "poisonous insect damage" in Chinese medicine. It is usually due to being stung or bitten by a bee, a mosquito, or a scorpion whereby the poisonous elements enter into the human body.

Alum & Young Tea Leaves Tea (*Ming Fan Ya Cha*)

Alumen (*Ming Fan*)   Equal amount
Young Tea leaves, *i.e.*, young Folium Camellia Theae (*Ya Cha*)   Equal amount

Method of administration: Grind the ingredients into a fine powder. Mix the powder with cold water and then spread it on the wound.

Functions: Clears heat and resolves toxins, stops itching and disperses swelling

Indications: This tea is suitable for the treatment of all mosquito and insect bites.

Contraindications: This formula is for external application only and should not be takin internally.

Clearing Tea (*Qing Cha*)

Tea leaves, *i.e.*, Folium Camelliae Theae (*Cha Ye*)   6 grams

Method of administration: Soak the Tea leaves in water. Use the Tea water to wash or spread on the wound.

Functions: Drains heat and resolves toxins

Indications: This tea is suitable for the treatment of different types of insect bite localized redness, swelling, and inflammation, extreme itching all over the body, heart vexation, and thirst.

Topically Applied Dampness Tea (*Wai Fu Shi Cha*)

Tea leaves, *i.e.*, Folium Camelliae Theae (*Cha Ye*)   A suitable amount

Method of administration: Soak the Tea leaves in water and then pound into pieces. Apply these topically to the affected area.

Functions: Resolves toxins, disperses swelling, and stops pain and itching

Indications: This tea is suitable for the topical application to bee stings and insect bites.

Spontaneous Sweating Teas

Spontaneous sweating means sweating not due to the use of diaphoretics or other stimulants and not due to strong exertion or excessive heat. Spontaneous sweating is mainly due to insecurity of the defensive qi and the qi's inability to secure fluids. Typically, defensive qi vacuity is due to heart, lung, spleen, and/or kidney qi and/or yang vacuities. After sweating, the body feels cold and the person feels fatigued.

Secure the Exterior Tea (*Gu Biao Cha*)

Radix Astragali Membranacei (*Huang Qi*)	12 grams
Radix Ledebouriellae Divaricatae (*Fang Feng*)	8 grams
Rhizoma Atractylodis Macrocephalae (*Bai Zhu*)	6 grams
Umeboshi, *i.e.*, Fructus Pruni Mume (*Wu Mei*)	5 grams

Method of administration: Place the above four herbs into a thermos, pour in boiling water, and soak for 15 minutes. Another method is to place the herbs into a pot and boil with water. Take 1 packet per day.

Functions: Boosts the qi and secures the exterior, stops sweating and allays thirst

Indications: This tea is suitable for the treatment of exterior vacuity spontaneous sweating and thirst. This formula is a good health drink for individuals with a weak constitution and excessive perspiration and who have a tendency to catch cold easily. It helps increase immunity and enables the body to become stronger and healthier. However, it should not be taken by a normal person as it may, in that case, only increase stagnation and depressive heat.

Astragalus & Red Date Tea (*Huang Qi Hong Zao Cha*)

Radix Astragali Membranacei (*Huang Qi*)	15 grams
Red dates, *i.e.*, Fructus Zizyphi Jujubae (*Hong Zao*)	5 pieces

Method of administration: Boil these two ingredients with water into a strong liquid. Drink this frequently at any time, 1 or 2 packets per day.

Functions: Fortifies the spleen and boosts the qi, regulates and harmonizes constructive and defense

Indications: This tea is suitable for the treatment of spontaneous sweating due to qi vacuity.

Contraindications: This tea is not suitable for copious perspiration due to a common cold or flu.

Wheat & Dioscorea Tea (*Xiao Mai Shan Yao Cha*)

Blighted wheat, *i.e.*, Semen Levis Tritici Aestivi (*Fu Xiao Mai*)	30 grams
Radix Dioscoreae Oppositae (*Shan Yao*)	32 grams

Method of administration: Place the blighted wheat in a cloth bag and boil with the dioscorea. Discard the dregs and use the liquid. Take 1 packet per day. Drink this as a tea.

Functions: Supplements vacuity and constrains perspiration

Indications: This tea is suitable for the treatment of spontaneous perspiration, night sweats, a thin body with lack of strength, getting flustered and short of breath easily, and restless sleep with profuse dreams.

Cornus Tea (*Shan Yu Rou Cha*)

Fructus Corni Officinalis (*Shan Zhu Yu*)	20 grams
Cortex Radicis Lycii Chinensis (*Di Gu Pi*)	3 grams
Radix Astragali Membranacei (*Huang Qi*)	3 grams

Method of administration: Grind the above three ingredients into a coarse powder. Place this powder in a cup. Pour boiling water over this powder, cover, and let steep for 15 minutes. Another method is to boil the herbs with water. Drink this continuously for 5 days, 1 packet per day.

Functions: Supplements vacuity, constrains and stops perspiration, clears heat, engenders fluid, and stops thirst

Indications: This tea is suitable for the treatment of spontaneous perspiration, night sweats, and thirsting and wasting.

Wheat & Rice Root Tea (*Xiao Mai Dao Gen Cha*)

Blighted wheat, *i.e.*, Semen Levis Tritici Aestivi (*Fu Xiao Mai*)   30 grams
Radix Et Rhizoma Oryzae Glutinosae (*Nuo Dao Gen*)   30 grams
Red dates, *i.e.*, Fructus Zizyphi Jujubae (*Da Zao*)   10 pieces

Method of administration: Boil these three ingredients in water twice. Discard the dregs and save the liquid. Drink this frequently at any time.

Functions: Supplements the qi and secures the exterior

Indications: This tea is suitable for treating qi vacuity and insecurity of the exterior causing spontaneous perspiration, a cold body, and chilled limbs.

Night Sweats Tea

Night sweats refers to sweating during sleep. This sweating stops upon awakening and there is no feeling of any aversion to cold. In fact, the opposite occurs, or, in other words, a feeling of vexatious heat. This is usually seen as due to yin vacuity with heat disturbing the heart. Thus fluids are unable to be constrained and stored. As it is stated in the *Nei Jing (Inner Classic)*, "If yang is greater than yin, it causes sweating." The treatment of this pattern, therefore, focuses primarily on nourishing yin and clearing heat.

Blighted Wheat & Ephedra Root Tea (*Fu Mai Ma Gen Cha*)

Blighted wheat, *i.e.*, Semen Levis Tritici Aestivi (*Fu Xiao Mai*)   30 grams
Radix Ephedrae (*Ma Huang Gen*)   6 grams

Method of administration: Grind these two ingredients into a coarse powder. Boil this powder with water and drink. Use 1 packet per day.

Functions: Supplements vacuity and nourishes the heart, constrains and stops sweating

Indications: This tea is suitable for the treatment of night sweats.

Facial Complexion Teas

The formulas in this section treat wrinkled skin, abnormal pigmentation, freckles, black or yellow-brown spots, and butterfly macules. In TCM, the causes of these conditions are liver/kidney depletion and detriment, blood vacuity lack of luster, or liver depression/qi stagnation. Taking the following tea formulas can often help to disperse spots, clean the facial surface, beautify the facial complexion, eliminate wrinkles, and combat skin aging.

Ci Xi's Pearl Tea (*Ci Xi Zhen Zhu Cha*)

Pearl, *i.e.*, Margarita (*Zhen Zhu*)	A suitable amount
Tea, *i.e.*, Folium Camelliae Theae (*Cha*)	A suitable amount

Note: Pearl powder can be purchased already prepared in small tubes at Chinese apothecaries in Chinatowns in large Western cities.

Method of administration: Choose sparkling or crystal clear, smooth, round pearls and grind them into a fine powder. Store this powder in a sealed porcelain pot. Make tea with boiled water and Tea leaves. Use 1 small spoonful of the pearl powder (2-3 grams) and drink with the Tea water. Drink warm, once every 10 days.

Functions: Lubricates the flesh and moistens the skin, preserves youth and beautifies the facial complexion

Indications: This tea is suitable for the treatment of facial skin aging.

Honey & Vinegar Fortify the Body Tea (*Mi Cu Jian Shen Cha*)

Cooking vinegar (*Shi Cu*)	15 grams
Honey (*Feng Mi*)	8 grams
Ginger juice, *i.e.,* Succus Rhizomatis Zingiberis (*Jiang Zhi*)	2 grams

Method of administration: Place these three ingredients in a cup and stir well. Pour in 5 times the amount of cool, boiled, *i.e.*, drinking water, stir well again, and drink. Use 1 packet per day.

Functions: Enriches and lubricates the skin, softens the blood vessels, lowers pressure, increases the appetite, disperses and eliminates fatigue

Indications: This tea is suitable for the treatment of dry skin, hypertension, fatigue, and aversion to food.

Clean the Face Tea (*Jing Mian Cha*)

Fructus Tribuli Terrestris (*Bai Ji Li*)	6 grams
Cortex Radicis Dictamni Dasycarpi (*Bai Xian Pi*)	6 grams
Radix Angelicae Sinensis (*Dang Gui*)	8 grams
Hawthorn fruit, *i.e.*, Fructus Crataegi (*Shan Zha*)	8 grams

Method of administration: Wash the above four herbs well. Place them in a cup and soak in boiling water. Use 1 packet per day.

Functions: Nourishes the blood and regulates the liver, resolves depression and dispels stasis

Indications: This tea is suitable for the treatment of yellow-brown spots on the skin, *i.e.*, chloasma or liver spots, especially postpartum or in women who take oral contraceptive pills.

Beautify the Face Tea (*Mei Yan Cha*)

Chinese olive, *i.e.*, Fructus Canarii (*Qing Guo*)	5 grams
Longan fruit, *i.e.*, Arillus Euphoriae Longanae (*Long Yan Rou*)	5 grams
Fructus Lycii Chinensis (*Gou Qi Zi*)	6 grams
Crystal sugar (*Bing Tang*)	Amount to taste

Method of administration: Wash the above three herbs well, place in a cup, and add the crystal sugar. Pour in boiling water and steep. Use 1 packet per day.

Functions: Nourishes the blood and enriches yin

Indications: This tea is suitable for beautifying the face and protecting the skin, especially in patients with yin vacuity and in thin individuals with lusterless skin. This formula has the effect of supplementing vacuity detriment, promotes the growth of flesh, and nourishes the complexion. Taken often, this tea encourages full and abundant qi and blood, a rosy complexion, energetic spirit, and lasting beauty.

Walnut & Milk Tea (*Hu Tao Niu Ru Cha*)

Walnut, *i.e.*, Semen Juglandis Regiae (*Hu Tao Rou*)	30 grams
Milk (*Niu Nai*)	180 grams
Soybean milk (*Dou Jiang*)	180 grams
Black sesame seeds, *i.e.*, black Semen Sesami Indici (*Hei Zhi Ma*)	20 grams
White sugar (*Bai Tang*)	Amount to taste
or Chicken egg (*Ji Dan*)	1 egg

Method of administration: One method is to mix the milk and soybean milk well, pour slowly into a container with the walnut and sesame seed, slowly grinding at the same time. After they are all well ground, pour into a pot and boil, adding in a small amount of sugar. Then drink it. Another method is to boil the milks, add the egg, and stir well. Take the first method 2 times per day, 1 bowl in the morning and 1 bowl in the evening. Using the latter method, take 1 bowl per day.

Functions: Nourishes the blood and lubricates the skin, dispels spots and engenders hair

Indications: This tea is suitable for the treatment of yellow-brown spots and loss of hair due to liver/kidney vacuity.

144

9
Male Reproductive Diseases

Impotence Teas

Impotence is the inability to achieve and/or maintain an erection sufficient to have sexual intercourse. In Western medicine, this may be due to anatomical or organic causes, mental or psychogenic disturbances, or poor health, medication, or paralysis. According to TCM, this condition may be due to masturbation at an early age, sexual hyperactivity, fear, fright, nervousness, chronic debility, or physical weakness.

Ginseng Strengthen Yang Tea (*Ren Shen Zhuang Yang Cha*)

Ginseng, *i.e.*, Radix Panacis Ginseng (*Ren Shen*)   9 grams
Tea leaves, *i.e.*, Folium Camelliae Theae (*Cha Ye*)   3 grams

Method of administration: Boil these two ingredients in 500ml of water. Take 1 packet per day, drunk warm.

Functions: Invigorates yang and supplements the source, strengthens the kidneys and boosts the qi

Indications: This tea is suitable for the treatment of impotence with no ejaculation or infirm erection and male sexual dysfunction.

Epimedium Tea (*Yin Yang Huo Cha*)

Herba Epimedii (*Yin Yang Huo*)   20 grams

Method of administration: Boil this herb or steep it in boiling water. Use 1 packet per day. Drink this as a tea over a long period of time.

Functions: Supplements the kidneys and invigorates yang

Indications: This tea is suitable for the treatment of impotence, premature ejaculation, seminal emission, and sexual neurosis.

Dried Shrimp Tea (*Xia Mi Cha*)

Dried shrimp (*Xia Mi*)   10 grams
White sugar (*Bai Tang*)   Amount to taste

Method of administration: Place the dried shrimp and white sugar in a cup, pour in boiling water, and cover for 5 minutes. Use 2 packets per day, taken in 2 separate doses.

Functions: Reinforces yang and lifts the spirit, nourishes, enriches, and supplements

Indications: This tea is suitable for the treatment of male impotence and cold sperm which is clear and scanty. It adds nutrition, maintains bodily functions, and increases immunity.

Walnut Instant Tea (*Hu Tao Su Rong Cha*)

Walnut, *i.e.*, Semen Juglandis Regiae (*Hu Tao Rou*)   500 grams
Lotus root starch (*Ou Fen*)   100 grams
White sugar (*Bai Tang*)   500 grams

Method of administration: Use fresh walnut and stir-fry over a gentle fire until slightly burned. Grind into a fine powder and mix this powder with the Lotus root starch and white sugar. Store for later use. Each time, use a few spoonfuls of the mixed powder. Pour boiling water over the powder, stirring at the same time. Drink this frequently as a tea.

Functions: Supplements the kidneys and lifts the spirit

Indications: This tea is suitable for the treatment of impotence.

Premature Ejaculation Teas

Premature ejaculation refers to ejaculation before penetration, upon penetration, or rapidly and involuntarily soon after penetration. In TCM, this is due to sexual hyperactivity or frequent masturbation that leads to kidney essence depletion and consumption, kidney yin insufficiency, and hyperactivity of ministerial fire, or weak constitution with marked emaciation, chronic vacuity detriment and seminal emission that leads to both kidney yin and kidney yang vacuities. In Chinese medicine, premature ejaculation and impotence have a close relationship. Severe premature ejaculation can cause impotence, and impotence often accompanies premature ejaculation.

Schisandra Tea (*Wu Wei Zi Cha*)

Fructus Schisandrae Chinensis (*Wu Wei Zi*)	10 grams
Crystal sugar (*Bing Tang*)	Amount to taste

Method of administration: Slightly heat the herb in hot water. Then pour boiling water over the herb, cover the cup for 5 minutes, and then add crystal sugar. Drink this freely as a tea.

Functions: Secures the essence and stops emission

Indications: This tea is suitable for the treatment of premature ejaculation, seminal emission, and neurasthenia.

Walnut Tea (*Tao Ren Cha*)

Walnut, *i.e.*, Semen Juglandis Regiae (*Hu Tao Rou*)	20 grams
White sugar (*Bai Tang*)	Amount to taste

Method of administration: Stir-fry the walnuts until cooked and then chop into pieces. Pour boiling water over the nuts and add the white sugar to taste. Drink this frequently as a tea.

Functions: Supplements the kidneys, strengthens and invigorates yang

Indications: This tea is suitable for the prevention of premature ejaculation.

Seminal Emission Teas

Seminal emission refers to the involuntary discharge of semen during sleep. In TCM, this is divided into the two types of dream emission and seminal efflux. Seminal emission that occurs during a dream is called dream emission. Emission that occurs without dreaming is called seminal efflux. If unmarried young men have seminal emission occasionally (1-2 times a month) with no discomfort or other symptoms, then this is considered a normal physiological phenomenon, not a pathological state, and no treatment is required. If the emissions occur fairly frequently with symptoms of a clouded head, tinnitus, sore low back, and lassitude of the spirit, then these tea formulas can be helpful.

Lotus Plumule Tea (*Lian Xin Cha*)

Plumula Nelumbinis Nuciferae (*Lian Xin*)	5 grams

Method of administration: Place the herb in a cup and steep in boiling water. Drink this at any time as a tea.

Functions: Clears the heart, drains heat, and secures the essence

Indications: This tea is suitable for the treatment of heart fire hyperactivity and exuberance, vexation of the heart, thirst, and seminal emission.

Astragalus Compalanatus Seed Tea (*Sha Yuan Ji Li Cha*)

Semen Astragali Complanati (*Sha Yuan Ji Li*)   10 grams

Method of administration: Wash the herb well and place in a teacup. Soak in boiling water. Use 1 packet per day and drink this frequently as a tea.

Functions: Supplements the kidneys and secures the essence, brightens the eyes and lightens the face

Indications: This tea is suitable for moistening the skin and retarding aging and for the treatment of kidney vacuity seminal emission and premature ejaculation.

Alpinia Oxyphylla Tea (*Yi Zhi Ren Cha*)

Black cardamon, *i.e.*, Fructus Alpiniae Oxyphyllae (*Yi Zhi Ren*)   50 grams
Alcohol (*Jiu*)   A suitable amount

Method of administration: Boil this herb with alcohol and water and then drink. Take once per day.

Functions: Warms the kidneys and stops emission

Indications: This tea is suitable for the treatment of insufficient kidney source qi and lower burner vacuity and coldness that are unable to restrain and control water and liquids, thus giving rise to the symptoms of enuresis, seminal emission, a cold body, and fear of the cold.

Leek Seed Tea (*Jiu Zi Cha*)

Chinese leek seeds, *i.e.*, Semen Allii Tuberosis (*Jiu Zi*)   20 grains
Salt (*Yan*)   A suitable amount

Method of administration: Boil this herb in salty water and drink it as a tea.

Functions: Nourishes yin and clears the heart, boosts the kidneys and secures the essence

Indications: This tea is suitable for the treatment of seminal emission due to chronic emotional problems affecting the kidneys. This condition is usually due to sexual fantasies that cause heart fire hyperactivity and exuberance.

Raspberry Tea (*Fu Pen Zi Cha*)

Raspberry, *i.e.*, Fructus Rubi (*Fu Pen Zi*)   15 grams
Green Tea, *i.e.*, Folium Camelliae Theae (*Lu Cha*)   A suitable amount

Method of administration: Steep these two ingredients in boiling water. Drink the resulting tea warm at any time.

Functions: Boosts the kidneys and secures the essence

Indications: This tea is suitable for the treatment of seminal emission, frequent urination, and impotence due to kidney qi vacuity not securing and astringing.

A Pair of Seeds Tea (*Shuang Ren Cha*)

Pinenut, *i.e.*, Semen Pini (*Song Zi Ren*)   15 grams
Walnut, *i.e.*, Semen Juglandis Regiae (*Hu Tao Rou*)   15 grams
Honey (*Feng Mi*)   15 grams

Method of administration: Steep these two seeds in boiling water for 10 minutes. Peel off their skins, pound them into a paste, add honey, and mix evenly. Use 10 grams each dose, taken with boiled water.

Functions: Secures the essence and supplements the blood

Indications: This tea is suitable for the treatment of seminal emission and premature ejaculation.

Mulberry & Sweet Water Beverage Tea (*Sang Shen Tang Shui Yin Cha*)

Fresh mulberry, *i.e.*, fresh Fructus Mori Albi (*Xian Sang Shen*)   60 grams
White or crystal sugar (*Bai Tang* or *Bing Tang*)   Amount to taste

Method of administration: Use fresh mulberries which are purple red in color. Boil with 2 bowls of clear water until only 1 bowl of liquid is left. Add the white sugar (or crystal sugar) to taste and drink the liquid after straining the dregs. Drink this as a tea frequently.

Functions: Supplements the liver and boosts the kidneys, nourishes yin and moistens dryness

Indications: This tea is suitable for the treatment of seminal emission, neurasthenia, and habitual constipation due to liver blood and kidney qi vacuity.

Cornus Tea (*Shan Zhu Yu Cha*)

Fructus Corni Officinalis (*Shan Zhu Yu*)   60 grams
Black cardamon, *i.e.*, Fructus Alpiniae Oxyphyllae (*Yi Zhi Ren*)   50 grams
Radix Codonopsitis Pilosulae (*Dang Shen*)   25 grams
Rhizoma Atractylodis Macrocephalae (*Bai Zhu*)   25 grams

Method of administration: Boil the above four ingredients in a pot with water and use the liquid. One packet may be used for 10 doses. Take 2 doses each day.

Functions: Warms and supplements the spleen and kidneys, secures the essence and reduces urination

Indications: This tea is suitable for the treatment of kidney vacuity with symptoms of seminal emission, impotence, sore low back and knees, and frequent urination. It is also good for the elderly with frequent urinary incontinence or constant vacuity sweating.

Low Sexual Desire Teas

Low sexual desire refers to sexual dysfunction that includes no desire for intercourse even with sexual stimulation, indifference toward intercourse, and difficulty in achieving erection. It often coexists with impotence.

Ginseng Tea (*Shen Cha*)

Ginseng, *i.e.*, Radix Panacis Ginseng (*Ren Shen*)	15 grams
Tea leaves, *i.e.*, Folium Camelliae Theae (*Cha Ye*)	5 grams

Method of administration: Boil the ginseng in water for 30 minutes. Then make tea with that liquid and Tea leaves. Drink this frequently. If the taste is too strong, add more boiled water until it is lighter.

Functions: Supplements the qi and assists yang

Indications: This tea is suitable for the treatment of kidney yang insufficiency, low sexual desire, impotence, lassitude of the spirit, fatigue, shortness of breath, disinclination to speak, fear of cold, cold limbs, and low back pain and weak legs. The tongue is pale and the pulse is deep and slow.

Lycium & Green Tea (*Qi Zi Lu Cha*)

Fructus Lycii Chinensis (*Gou Qi Zi*)   15 grams
Green Tea, *i.e.*, Folium Camelliae Theae (*Lu Cha*)   3 grams

Method of administration: Place these two ingredients in a teacup and pour boiling water into the cup. Drink this frequently while still hot. Use 1 packet per day taken as a tea.

Functions: Boosts the liver and brightens the eyes, supplements the kidneys and moistens the lungs

Indications: This tea is suitable for the treatment of liver/kidney insufficiency with decreased sexual desire, low back and knee soreness and weakness, tidal fever and night sweating, and dizziness and tinnitus.

Carrot Tea (*Hu Luo Bo Cha*)

Carrot (*Hu Luo Bo*)   150 grams
Apple (*Ping Guo*)   200 grams
Cow's milk (*Niu Nai*)   100 ml
Chicken egg yolk (*Ji Dan Huang*)   1 yolk
Ginseng wine (*Ren Shen Jiu*)   30 ml
Honey (*Feng Mi*)   A suitable amount

Note: See *Chinese Medicinal Wines & Elixirs* by Bob Flaws, Blue Poppy Press, Boulder, CO, 1995 for instructions on how to make ginseng wine.

Method of administration: Chop the hard ingredients into small pieces. Place these together with the liquid ingredients into a blender and puree. Cold water may be added if desired. Drink this daily as a tea.

Functions: Enriches, supplements, strengthens, and invigorates

Indications: This tea is suitable for the treatment of low sexual desire and impotence.

Sterility Teas

Sterility is to men what infertility is to women. Except for a few cases which are due to organic pathological change, it is usually a functional problem. This problem includes seminal emission, premature ejaculation, impotence, no viable semen, seminal blockage, scanty spermatozoa with low motility, chronic spermatozoa liquefaction or no liquefaction, no spermatozoa, and reproductive organ inflammation. Clinically, different types of symptoms often coexist. Teas should be chosen based on a TCM pattern discrimination.

Cuscutae Tea (*Tu Si Zi Cha*)

Semen Cuscutae (*Tu Si Zi*)	10 grams
Brown sugar (*Hong Tang*)	Amount to taste

Method of administration: Rinse the herb well, pound it to pieces, and add the brown sugar. Steep in boiling water and drink as a tea.

Functions: Supplements the kidneys and secures the essence

Indications: This tea is suitable for the treatment of a low sperm count, premature ejaculation, and low back and knee soreness and weakness.

Five Seed Supplement the Kidneys Tea (*Wu Zi Bu Shen Cha*)

Semen Cuscutae (*Tu Si Zi*)	250 grams
Fructus Lycii Chinensis (*Gou Qi Zi*)	250 grams
Raspberry, *i.e.*, Fructus Rubi (*Fu Pen Zi*)	125 grams
Plantain seed, *i.e.*, Semen Plantaginis (*Che Qian Zi*)	60 grams
Fructus Schisandrae Chinensis (*Wu Wei Zi*)	30 grams

Method of administration: Grind the herbs together into a fine powder. Use 9-12 grams of the resulting powder each time. Steep in boiling water and drink this as a tea. Take 2 packets per day.

Functions: Supplements the kidneys and boosts the essence, supports yang, secures and astringes

Indications: This tea is suitable for the treatment of male sterility and female infertility with the symptoms of seminal emission, impotence, premature ejaculation, or endless dribbling after urination. Clinical experience shows that by adding 250 grams of Deer Antler, *i.e.*, Cornu Parvum Cervi (*Lu Rong*), and 250 grams of Mantis Egg Case, *i.e.*, Ootheca Mantidis (*Sang Piao Xiao*), to the above formula, there are fairly good results for abnormal sperm and a low survival rate of the sperms affecting reproductive ability. Generally, this formula needs to be taken for at least 3 months to 6 months.

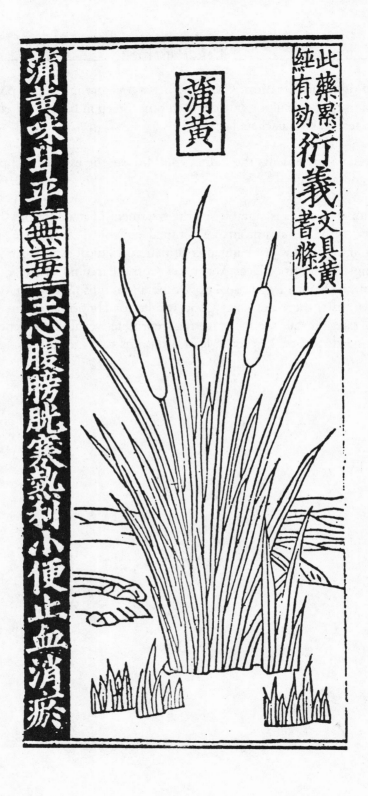

蒲黄

此藥累文具黃
絲有勁
衍義
書絛下

蒲黃味甘平無毒主心腹膀胱寒熱利小便止血消瘀

10
Gynecological & Obstetrical Diseases

Excessive Menstruation Teas

If menstrual cycle is normal but the amount of the menses is excessive, this is referred to as excessive menstruation. Commonly, excessive menstruation and early menstruation occur together since both are, in a sense, types of pathological bleeding which share common causes.

Lotus Seed Tea (*Lian Zi Cha*)

Tea leaves, *i.e.*, Folium Camelliae Theae (*Cha Ye*)	5 grams
Lotus seed, *i.e.*, Semen Nelumbinis Nuciferae (*Lian Zi*)	30 grams
Crystal sugar (*Bing Tang*)	20 grams

Method of administration: Soak the Tea leaves in boiling water and then use only the liquid. Soak the lotus seeds in warm water for a few hours. Then stew them with the crystal sugar, add the Tea water, and stir well. Remove the dregs and drink as a tea.

Functions: Fortifies the spleen and boosts the kidneys

Indications: This tea is suitable for the treatment of excessive menstruation or constant uterine bleeding and vaginal discharge due to combination of qi vacuity not astringing and heat causing the blood to move recklessly or frenetically.

Black Wood Ear & Red Date Tea (*Hei Mu Er Hong Zao Cha*)

Black wood ear, *i.e.,* Exidia Auricula Judae (*Hei Mu Er*)   30 grams
Red dates, *i.e.,* Fructus Zizyphi Jujubae (*Hong Zao*)   20 pieces

Method of administration: Boil these two ingredients, remove the dregs, and reserve the liquid. Take 1 time per day. Drink this tea continuously for some time.

Functions: Supplements the middle and boosts the qi, nourishes blood and stops bleeding

Indications: This tea is suitable for the treatment of a weak constitution, anemia, excessive menstruation, and hemorrhoidal bleeding due to spleen qi vacuity.

Artemisia Apiacea & Moutan Tea (*Qing Hao Dan Pi Cha*)

Herba Artemisiae Apiaceae (*Qing Hao*)   6 grams
Tree peony root bark, *i.e.,* Cortex Radicis Moutan (*Dan Pi*)   6 grams
Tea leaves, *i.e.,* Folium Camelliae Theae (*Cha Ye*)   3 grams
Crystal sugar (*Bing Tang*)   15 grams

Method of administration: Wash the first two ingredients well. Place the three herbs in a teacup and soak in just boiled water for 15-20 minutes. Add the crystal sugar and allow it to dissolve. Use 1 packet per day. Drink as a tea.

Functions: Clears heat, cools the blood, and stops bleeding

Indications: This tea is suitable for the treatment of early menstruation or for two menstrual periods within one month where the flow is copious in quantity with a purple color and is sticky and thick in consistency. It is also for vexatious heat of the heart and chest with reddish yellow urine and a fishy and foul white vaginal discharge. The tongue is red with a thick, yellow coating.

The pulse is strong and rapid. Thus this tea is indicated for blood heat and damp heat patterns.

Brown Sugar Strong Tea (*Hong Tang Nong Cha*)

Rhizoma Imperatae Cylindricae (*Bai Mao Gen*)	10 grams
Tea leaves, *i.e.*, Folium Camelliae Theae (*Cha Ye*)	A suitable amount
Brown sugar (*Hong Tang*)	A suitable amount

Method of administration: Boil the herbal ingredients into 1 bowl of strong liquid. Strain off the dregs and add in the brown sugar, allowing it to dissolve. Drink this twice a day.

Functions: Clears heat and regulates menstruation

Indications: This tea is suitable for the treatment of early menstruation with copious blood flow due to blood heat.

Scanty Menstruation Teas

Scanty menstruation is a TCM term for a shorter than normal menstrual period (usually only 1-2 days) or a regular menstrual period with very little blood (usually 30ml or less). Both symptoms usually appear together and may be premonitory symptoms to "menstrual block" or amenorrhea.

Regulate Menstruation Tea (*Tiao Jing Cha*)

Radix Angelica Sinensis (*Dang Gui*)	60 grams
Radix Ligustici Wallichii (*Chuan Xiong*)	10 grams
Motherwort, *i.e.*, Herba Leonuri Heterophylli (*Yi Mu Cao*)	45 grams

Method of administration: Rinse the herbs and then boil them in water. Use 1 packet per day and drink the resulting liquid as a tea. The same packet may be boiled repeatedly.

Functions: Regulates the menstruation, quickens the blood, and stops pain

Indications: This tea is suitable for the treatment of irregular menstruation with decreased flow, abdominal pain during menstruation, delayed menstruation, or postpartum abdominal pain due to blood stasis possibly, but not necessarily, complicated by blood vacuity.

Black Soybean & Sappan Wood Tea (*Hei Dou Su Mu Cha*)

Black soybeans, *i.e.*, black Semen Glycinis (*Hei Dou*)   100 grams
Lignum Sappan (*Su Mu*)   10 grams
Brown sugar (*Hong Tang*)   Amount to taste

Method of administration: Stew the first two ingredients with water until the black soybeans are thoroughly cooked. Remove the sappan wood, add the brown sugar, and allow it to dissolve. Take 2 doses per day, drinking the liquid *and* eating the black soybeans.

Functions: Supplements the kidneys and quickens the blood

Indications: This tea is suitable to take during the latter part of the menstruation if the amount of menstrual flow has been scanty due to a combination of blood vacuity and blood stasis.

Motherwort Tea (*Yi Mu Cao Cha*)

Motherwort, *i.e.*, Herba Leonuri Heterophylli (*Yi Mu Cao*)   60 grams
Brown sugar (*Hong Tang*)   50 grams

Method of administration: Place the herb in a pot and boil with 200ml of water. Discard the dregs, add the brown sugar, and allow it to dissolve. Drink this liquid immediately. After drinking, place a hot water bottle (or similar device) on the abdomen to warm the area.

Functions: Quickens the blood and regulates menstruation

Indications: This tea is suitable for the treatment of very small amounts of menstrual blood which, in the worst cases, are only drops of blood or for excessively short menstruation due to blood stasis.

Dysfunctional Uterine Bleeding Teas

Dysfunctional uterine bleeding is usually due to ovarian dysfunction without any organic pathological change to the uterus. Its symptoms are an irregular menstrual cycle, prolonged menstruation with an increased amount of flow, and a large, sudden onset of bleeding or dribbling, continual flow. In TCM, this condition belongs to the category of "flooding & leaking."

Agrimony Tea (*Xian He Cao Cha*)

Herba Agrimoniae Pilosae (*Xian He Cao*)   60 grams
Shepherd's purse, *i.e.*, Herba Capsellae Bursa-pastoris (*Ji Cai*)   50 grams

Method of administration: Rinse the two ingredients and place in a pot. Boil with water. Use 1 packet per day, drunk as a tea.

Functions: Stops bleeding and fortifies the stomach

Indications: This tea is suitable for the treatment of uterine bleeding and profuse menstrual flow due to heat.

Umeboshi & Brown Sugar Tea (*Wu Mei Hong Tang Cha*)

Umeboshi, *i.e.*, Fructus Pruni Mume (*Wu Mei*)   9 grams

Brown sugar (*Hong Tang*)   Amount to taste

Method of administration: Boil these two ingredients in 1 bowl of clear water until half a bowl is left. Strain off the dregs and drink as a warm tea twice a day.

Functions: Promotes contraction and stops bleeding

Indications: This tea is suitable for the treatment of dysfunctional uterine bleeding due to loss of securing and astringing.

Large or Small Thistle Instant Tea (*Da Ji Xiao Ji Su Rong Cha*)

Fresh Herba Cirsii Japonici (*Xian Da Ji*)
or fresh Herba Cephalonoplos Segeti (*Xian Xiao Ji*)   2500 grams
White sugar (*Bai Tang*)   500 grams

Method of administration: Wash the fresh thistle well and chop into pieces. Add a suitable amount of water and boil for 1 hour over a medium fire. Strain off the dregs and concentrate the liquid longer over a gentle fire. Remove from the heat and add the white sugar to absorb the liquid. Let cool and dry. Grind into powder and store. Using 10 grams each time, pour boiling water over the powder and allow to steep. The resulting tea may be taken 3-4 times a day.

Functions: Cools the blood and stops bleeding

Indications: This tea is suitable for the treatment of dysfunctional uterine bleeding due to heat.

Menstrual Pain Teas

Before, during, or after menstruation, pain may occur in the lower abdomen and sacral area. If the condition is severe, it may also be accompanied by headache, nausea, vomiting, diarrhea, heaviness, or a clouding inversion affecting life and work. Simply called "menstrual pain" in Chinese medicine, this usually occurs in young females and is one of the most commonly seen conditions in gynecology. It is usually divided into two types. Primary dysmenorrhea is pain that occurs at the initial stage of menstruation without pathological change in the pelvic cavity. Secondary dysmenorrhea is pain caused by organic pathological changes, such as edeitis, tumors, and endometriosis. Slight abdominal pain and mild discomfort in the sacral area during menstruation are considered normal.

Menstrual Pain Tea (*Tong Jing Cha*)

Rhizoma Cyperi Rotundi (*Xiang Fu*)	10 grams
Radix Linderae Strychnifoliae (*Wu Yao*)	10 grams
Rhizoma Corydalis Yanhusuo (*Yan Hu Suo*)	10 grams
Cinnamon bark, *i.e.*, Cortex Cinnamomi (*Rou Gui*)	3 grams

Method of administration: Grind the above herbs into powder and steep in boiling water. Use 1 packet per day and take continuously for 3-5 days.

Functions: Warms the channels, rectifies the qi, and stops pain

Indications: This tea is suitable for the treatment of dull pain in the lower abdomen, sometimes with distention and a full sensation or sometimes with a cold sensation in the lower abdomen. The pain and distention feel more comfortable with the application of heat either before or during menstruation.

Leonurus Tea (*Yi Mu Cao Cha*)

Dry motherwort, *i.e.*, dry Herba Leonuri Heterophylli (*Gan Pin Yi Mu Cao*)	20 grams
Green Tea, *i.e.*, Folium Camelliae Theae (*Lu Cha*)	1 gram

Method of administration: Place these two ingredients in a cup and steep in boiling water. Cover for 5 minutes and drink when the menstrual pain occurs.

Functions: Quickens the blood and regulates menstruation, lowers (blood) pressure and disinhibits water, stimulates the nerves

Indications: This tea is suitable for the treatment of primary dysmenorrhea associated with a pattern of blood stasis.

Lycopus Tea (*Ze Lan Cha*)

Dry Herba Lycopi Lucidi (*Gan Pin Ze Lan*)   10 grams
Green Tea, *i.e.*, Folium Camelliae Theae (*Lu Cha*)   1 gram

Method of administration: Place the above two ingredients in a cup and steep in boiling water. Cover the cup for 5 minutes and then drink as a tea at any time.

Functions: Quickens the blood and dispels stasis, frees menstruation and disinhibits the urine, fortifies the stomach and soothes the qi

Indications: This tea is suitable for the treatment of early or late periods with varying amounts of menstrual blood, and distention and pain in the lower abdomen due to qi stagnation and blood stasis.

Ligusticum Regulate Menstruation Tea (*Chuan Xiong Tiao Jing Cha*)

Radix Ligustici Wallichii (*Chuan Xiong*)   3 grams
Green Tea, *i.e.*, Folium Camelliae Theae (*Lu Cha*)   6 grams

Method of administration: Boil these two ingredients in 300-400ml of water until half (150-200ml) of the liquid is left. Take 1-2 packets per day, drinking it warm before meals.

Functions: Quickens the blood and dispels stasis, moves the qi and stops pain

Indications: This tea is suitable for the treatment of irregular menstruation, menstrual pain, menstrual block or amenorrhea, postpartum abdominal pain, and chest *bi* heart pain due to qi stagnation and blood stasis, as well as for wind heat headache.

Two Flowers Regulate Menstruation Tea (*Er Hua Tiao Jing Cha*)

Rose flower, *i.e.*, Flos Rosae Rugosae (*Mei Gui Hua*)	9 grams
Flos Et Fructus Rosae Chinensis (*Yue Ji Hua*)	9 grams
Black Tea, *i.e.*, prepared Folium Camelliae Theae (*Hong Cha*)	3 grams

Method of administration: Grind the above three ingredients into a coarse powder, steep in boiling water, and cover for 10 minutes. Use 1 packet per day. Drink this tea warm at any time continuously for a few days. It is beneficial to take this formula a few days before the menses begin.

Functions: Quickens the blood and regulates menstruation, rectifies the qi and stops pain

Indications: This tea is suitable for the treatment of qi stagnation and blood stasis which causes menstrual pain with a small amount of blood, abdominal distention and pain, dark-colored blood possibly with clots, or menstrual block, *i.e.*, amenorrhea.

Chinese Tea Rose Tea (*Yue Ji Hua Cha*)

Fresh Flos Et Fructus Rosae Chinensis (*Xian Yue Ji Hua*)	15-20 grams

Method of administration: Steep this herb in boiling water. Use 1 packet per day, taken continuously for a few days.

Functions: Quickens the blood and regulates menstruation

Indications: This tea is suitable for the treatment of irregular menstruation and abdominal pain during the period due to blood stasis. It can also be used for impact injury with pain.

Mugwort & Sugar Tea (*Ai Ye Tang Cha*)

Mugwort, *i.e.*, Folium Artemisiae Argyii (*Ai Ye*)	20 grams
Brown sugar (*Hong Tang*)	15 grams

Method of administration: Boil these two ingredients in water and drink as a tea.

Functions: Warms the channels and dispels cold and dampness

Indications: This tea is suitable for the treatment of cold damp congelation and stagnation menstrual pain. This is usually due to cold and damp damage reaching the *chong* and *ren* and the uterus. Cold congeals the qi and blood, causing lower abdominal chilly or gripping pain that decreases with heat, dark-colored blood with clots, and unsmooth menstruation.

Hawthorn & Sunflower Seed Tea (*Shan Zha Kui Zi Cha*)

Hawthorn fruit, *i.e.*, Fructus Crataegi (*Shan Zha*)	50 grams
Sunflower seeds (*Kui Hua Zi Ren*)	50 grams
Brown sugar (*Hong Tang*)	100 grams

Method of administration: Add water to the above three ingredients and stew into a soup. Take 1 packet a day in 2 divided doses. For best results, take this formula 2-3 days before the period.

Functions: Fortifies the spleen and stomach, supplements the middle, and boosts qi

Indications: This tea is suitable for the treatment of qi and blood vacuity menstrual pain.

Brown Sugar Tea (*Hong Tang Cha*)

Brown sugar (*Hong Tang*)	8 grams
Blast-fried ginger, *i.e.*, blast-fried Rhizoma Zingiberis (*Pao Jiang*)	3 grams
Tea leaves, *i.e.*, Folium Camelliae Theae (*Cha Ye*)	2 grams

Method of administration: Place these three ingredients in a cup and steep in boiling water for 1 minute. Drink this as a tea.

Functions: Supplements the middle and relaxes the liver, quickens the blood and dispels stasis, scatters cold and soothes the sinews

Indications: This tea is suitable for the treatment of lower abdominal cold pain and menstrual pain.

Amenorrhea Teas

Amenorrhea is called "menstrual block" in TCM. Menstrual block indicates that the menstruation is blocked and its absence is not due to menopause. Menstrual block is divided roughly into vacuity and repletion types. For the vacuity type, the treatment principles are to supplement and boost the qi and blood. For the repletion type, the treatment principles are to quicken the blood, dispel stasis, and free the channels.

Salvia & Sugar Tea (*Dan Shen Tang Cha*)

Radix Salviae Miltiorrhizae (*Dan Shen*)	60 grams
Brown sugar (*Hong Tang*)	60 grams

Method of administration: Boil these two ingredients in water and use the liquid. Take as a tea. Use 1 packet per day in 2 divided doses, once in the morning and once in the evening.

Functions: Quickens the blood and dispels stasis, nourishes the blood and regulates menstruation

Indications: This tea is suitable for the treatment of menstrual block due to yin blood insufficiency with the sea of blood empty and vacuous. The color of the blood is pale yellow, the spirit is tired, and there may be dizziness and tinnitus.

Rubia Tea (*Qian Cao Cha*)

Radix Rubiae Cordifoliae (*Qian Cao Gen*)   60 grams

Method of administration: Boil this herb in water. Use 1 packet per day, taken in 2 divided doses.

Functions: Quickens the blood and dispels stasis, moves the qi and resolves depression

Indications: This tea is suitable for the treatment of menstrual block due to qi stagnation and blood stasis, liver qi depression and binding, and blood moving unsmoothly, thus causing symptoms of depression, vexation, easy anger, chest and epigastric distention and oppression, distention in the lower abdomen, and distention and pain in the two coastal regions.

Ginger, Red Date & Brown Sugar Tea (*Jiang Zao Hong Tang Cha*)

Dry ginger, *i.e.*, dry Rhizoma Zingiberis (*Gan Jiang*)   30 grams
Red dates, *i.e.*, Fructus Zizyphi Jujubae (*Da Zao*)   30 grams
Brown sugar (*Hong Tang*)   30 grams

Method of administration: Clean the red dates and remove and discard the pits. Rinse the dry ginger and chop into slices. Add these two herbs to the brown sugar and boil. Use 1 packet per day, drunk warm in 2 doses.

Functions: Supplements the spleen and stomach, warms the middle, and boosts the qi

Indications: This tea is suitable for the treatment of menstrual pain due to cold damp congelation and stagnation or to qi and blood vacuity.

Vaginal Discharge Teas

Vaginal discharge refers to an abnormal, sticky vaginal discharge that is perpetual and incessant. In TCM, this is due to various disease mechanisms. The color of the discharge may be white, yellow, or red depending on these different disease mechanisms. In Western medicine, this is usually seen in vaginitis (mycotic trichomona) or cervicitis (endometrial inflammation).

Celosia Flower Tea (*Ji Guan Hua Cha*)

Celosia flower, *i.e.*, Flos Celesiae Cristatae (*Ji Guan Hua*)   30 grams

Method of administration: Chop the herb into pieces and boil with water. Use 1 packet per day. Drink the resulting liquid frequently as a tea.

Functions: Astringes and stops discharge

Indications: This tea is suitable for the treatment of red and white discharge. It is known to be able to kill vaginal trichomonads.

Gingko Free Strangury Tea (*Bai Guo Tong Lin Cha*)

Semen Ginkgonis Bilobae (*Bai Guo*)   50 grams
Chinese wax gourd seed, *i.e.*, Semen Benincasae Hispidae
   (*Dong Gua Zi*)   25 grams

169

Lotus seed, *i.e.*, Semen Nelumbinis Nuciferae (*Lian Zi*)   20 grams
Powdered black pepper, *i.e.*, powdered Fructus Piperis Nigri
   (*Hu Jiao Fen*)   15 grams
White sugar (*Bai Tang*)   Amount to taste

Method of administration: Remove the skin and heart of the ginkgo nut and dispose of the middle of the lotus seed. Then boil these two herbs with the wax gourd seed and water in a pot for 40 minutes and filter the decoction. Using the remaining liquid, add the pepper powder and white sugar and mix well. Drink this as a tea.

Functions: Fortifies the spleen and supplements the kidneys, frees strangury and stops discharge

Indications: This tea is suitable for the treatment of white discharge and turbid strangury due to dampness and heat but more dampness than heat.

Hyacinth Bean & Dioscorea Tea (*Bian Dou Shan Yao Cha*)

Hyacinth bean, *i.e.*, Semen Dolichoris Lablab (*Bai Bian Dou*)   20 grams
Radix Dioscoreae Oppositae (*Shan Yao*)   20 grams
White sugar (*Bai Tang*)   Amount to taste

Method of administration: Stir-fry the hyacinth beans until they are yellowish and then pound into pieces. Next, slice the dioscorea. Boil these two herbs together. Using the remaining liquid, add the sugar and let it dissolve. Use 1 packet per day. Drink frequently as a tea.

Functions: Fortifies the spleen and dries dampness

Indications: This tea is suitable for the treatment of spleen vacuity discharge, *i.e.*, a white-colored discharge with other signs and symptoms of spleen vacuity, such as fatigue, lack of appetite, loose stools, etc.

Cistanches Tea (*Rou Cong Rong Cha*)

Herba Cistanchis Deserticolae (*Rou Cong Rong*)   20 grams

Method of administration: Boil this herb in water. Use 1 packet per day taken in 2 divided doses. Take it once in the morning and once in the evening.

Functions: Warms yang and supplements the kidneys

Indications: This tea is suitable for the treatment of kidney vacuity white discharge. In TCM his is usually due to an early marriage or multiple births that injure and damage kidney qi and causes a discharge that is copious in amount, clear and watery in consistency, dribbles constantly, and is accompanied by severe low back pain.

Pomegranate Tea (*Shi Liu Cha*)

Pomegranate peel, *i.e.*, Pericarpium Punicae Granati (*Shi Liu Pi*)   30 grams

Method of administration: Boil this herb in water and drink the resulting liquid as a tea.

Functions: Warms the kidneys and secures the vessels

Indications: This tea is suitable for the treatment of a vaginal discharge that is due to spleen and kidney vacuity or the *ren mai* not being secure/not securing. The discharge is white and sticky and is accompanied by low back and abdominal pain.

Stirring Fetus Teas

Stirring fetus is a disease category within TCM which roughly corresponds to threatened abortion. It is characterized by low back pain and sagging and distention in the lower abdomen accompanied by a small amount of vaginal bleeding during pregnancy. In TCM gynecology, there are also the categories of "fetal leakage" and "lower abdominal pain during pregnancy." In fetal leakage, there is vaginal bleeding during pregnancy but no low back or abdominal pain. In lower abdominal pain during pregnancy, there is abdominal pain but no bleeding. Stirring fetus is a combination of both these two and is a more ominous sign during pregnancy requiring speedy treatment. The main causes of stirring fetus are liver/kidney insufficiency, qi and blood vacuity, blood heat, blood stasis, and traumatic injury.

Walnut Tea (*Hu Tao Cha*)

Walnut, *i.e.*, Semen Juglandis Regiae (*Hu Tao Ren*)   10 nuts

Method of administration: Break the walnuts and boil, including the shells, in water. Remove the dregs and drink the liquid as a tea at any time. Use 1-2 packets per day.

Functions: Supplements the liver and kidneys and calms the fetus

Indications: This tea is suitable for the treatment of stirring fetus, low back pain, or hiccough.

Lotus Seed & Raisin Tea (*Lian Zi Pu Tao Gan Cha*)

Lotus seed, *i.e.*, Semen Nelumbinis Nuciferae (*Lian Zi*)   90 grams
Raisins, *i.e.*, dry Fructus Vitis Viniferae (*Pu Tao Gan*)   30 grams

Method of administration: Discard the skin and core of the lotus seeds. Wash them well and place together with the raisins in 700-800ml of water in a double boiler. Use a high fire to stew until the lotus seeds are well cooked. Take 1 time per day. The effects of this tea will be seen after taking 5-10 times.

Functions: Supplements the qi, boosts the liver, and calms the fetus

Indications: This tea is suitable for the treatment of stirring fetus due to qi and blood vacuity.

Sweet Rice & Astragalus Tea (*Nuo Mi Huang Qi Cha*)

Polished glutinous rice, *i.e.*, Semen Oryzae Glutinosae (*Nuo Mi*)   30 grams
Radix Astragali Membranacei (*Huang Qi*)   15 grams
Radix Ligustici Wallichii (*Chuan Xiong*)   5 grams

Method of administration: Boil these three ingredients in 1,000ml of water until only 500ml are left. Strain off the dregs and drink the liquid warm as a tea. Take 1 packet a day in 2 doses.

Functions: Regulates qi and blood and calms the fetus

Indications: This tea is suitable for the treatment of qi and blood vacuity stirring fetus.

Habitual Miscarriage Tea

In TCM, habitual miscarriage is most often called "slippery fetus." This refers to 3 or more consecutive natural miscarriages. It is usually due to qi vacuity, kidney vacuity, blood heat, or external injury causing each pregnancy to end in miscarriage.

Tender Corn Husk Tea (*Yu Mi Nen Yi Cha*)

Tender corn husk, *i.e.*, the inner-most tender husks (*Yu Mi Nen Yi*)   1 husk

Method of administration: Chop the tender husk into pieces and boil in water. Drink this frequently as a tea. Begin drinking this tea at the beginning of pregnancy until past the date of the last miscarriage. At that time, double the amount of the doses and continue drinking this amount until delivery.

Functions: Clears heat, disinhibits the urine, and secures the fetus

173

Indications: This tea is suitable for the treatment of habitual miscarriage due to blood heat.

Nausea & Vomiting During Pregnancy Teas

Nausea and vomiting during pregnancy are called morning sickness by lay people. This refers to the symptoms of nausea, vomiting, dizziness, aversion to food, or even vomiting right after eating during the first trimester of pregnancy. It is usually due to the qi of the *chong mai* counterflowing upward, thus causing impaired harmonious downbearing of the stomach.

Perilla Leaf & Fresh Ginger Tea (*Su Ye Sheng Jiang Cha*)

Perilla leaf, *i.e.*, Folium Perillae Frutescentis (*Zi Su Ye*)   4.5 grams
Fresh ginger juice, *i.e.*, Succus Rhizomatis Zingiberis
   (*Sheng Jiang Zhi*)   A few drops

Method of administration: Rub the perilla leaves into pieces. Steep them and the ginger juice in boiling water. Drink this tea frequently.

Functions: Rectifies the qi, harmonizes the stomach, and calms the fetus

Indications: This tea is suitable for the treatment of relatively light morning sickness due to loss of harmony of the stomach qi.

Coptis & Perilla Leaf Tea (*Huang Lian Su Ye Cha*)

Rhizoma Coptidis Chinensis (*Huang Lian*)   1.5 grams
Perilla leaf, *i.e.*, Folium Perillae Frutescentis (*Zi Su Ye*)   3 grams

Method of administration: Boil these two ingredients in water. Drink the resulting liquid as a tea repeatedly.

Functions: Clears heat and harmonizes the stomach

174

Indications: This tea is suitable for the treatment of vomiting during pregnancy due to depressive heat with loss of harmony of the stomach qi.

Sugarcane & Fresh Ginger Tea (*Gan Zhe Sheng Jiang Cha*)

Sugarcane juice (*Gan Zhe Zhi*)   10 grams
Fresh ginger juice, *i.e.*, Succus Rhizomatis Zingiberis (*Sheng Jiang Zhi*)   10 grams

Method of administration: Mix these two juices together and drink a small amount periodically throughout the day.

Functions: Fortifies the spleen and stomach and stops vomiting

Indications: This tea is suitable for the treatment of vomiting during pregnancy due to spleen vacuity.

Tangerine Peel & Bamboo Shavings Tea (*Ju Pi Zhu Ru Cha*)

Tangerine peel, *i.e.*, Pericarpium Citri Reticulatae (*Ju Pi*)   5 grams
Caulis Bambusae In Taeniis (*Zhu Ru*)   10 grams

Method of administration: Tear the tangerine peel into pieces. Chop the bamboo shavings into pieces. Steep both herbs in boiling water and repeatedly drink as a tea.

Functions: Clears heat and rectifies the qi, harmonizes the stomach and stops vomiting

Indications: This tea is suitable for the treatment of morning sickness due to stomach qi counterflowing upward complicated by depressive heat.

Postpartum Disease Teas

In TCM, injury during childbirth, postpartum hemorrhage, and damage to the original qi can cause "hundred of joints emptiness" postpartum. In addition, malnutrition and careless health preservation can easily create different postpartum diseases. Examples of postpartum diseases described in and treated by TCM gynecology are postpartum abdominal pain, postpartum blood dizziness, postpartum tetany, postpartum headache, postpartum constipation, postpartum dysentery, postpartum sweating, nipple inversion, and insufficient lactation. Postpartum diseases are usually due to vacuity and/or stasis. When treating postpartum diseases, it is very important to distinguish vacuity from repletion. Once these are differentiated, vacuity should be supplemented and repletion should be drained.

Brown Sugar & Black Pepper Tea (*Hong Tang Hu Jiao Cha*)

Brown sugar (*Hong Tang*)	15 grams
Black pepper, *i.e.*, Fructus Piperis Nigri (*Hu Jiao*)	1.5 grams
Black Tea, *i.e.*, prepared Folium Camelliae Theae (*Hong Cha*)	3 grams

Method of administration: Grind the black pepper into powder. Stir-fry this with the brown sugar until burnt. Steep this mixture with the Tea boiled in water. Take 1-2 packets per day.

Functions: Warms the middle, transforms stagnation, and stops dysentery

Indications: This tea is suitable for the treatment of postpartum dysentery with abdominal pain.

Cattail Pollen Tea (*Pu Huang Cha*)

Cattail pollen, *i.e.*, Pollen Typhae (*Pu Huang*)	100 grams

Method of administration: Boil the above herb in water. Drink it as a tea.

176

Functions: Quickens the blood and dispels stasis

Indications: This tea is suitable for the treatment of postpartum heart oppression and clouding inversion, *i.e.*, faintness and syncope, due to retention of the lochia and internal static blood that attacks upward injuring the heart and lungs.

Honey & Angelica Dahurica Tea (*Mi Zhi Cha*)

Radix Angelicae Dahuricae (*Bai Zhi*)	A suitable amount
Honey (*Feng Mi*)	A suitable amount
Tea leaves, *i.e.*, Folium Camelliae Theae (*Cha Ye*)	A suitable amount

Method of administration: Wash the angelica dahurica, dry, and grind into powder. Make this powder into balls about bullet size with the honey. Let the balls dry in a cool, airy place or dry with low heat. Store the dry balls in a sealed container for later use. Take 1 ball 2-3 times per day. It may be chewed or one can make tea from 6 grams of Tea leaves and then boil the ball in the liquid.

Functions: Dispels wind and resolves the exterior, rectifies the qi and stops pain

Indications: This tea is suitable for the treatment of women either during pregnancy or postpartum for wind damage headache, blood vacuity headache, or head wind dizziness.

Scallion Juice Tea (*Cong Xian Ti Hao Cha*)

Scallion juice, *i.e.,* Succus Allii Fistulosi (*Cong Xian*)	A suitable amount
Powdered Tea leaves, *i.e.*, powdered Folium Camelliae Theae (*Cha Ye Mo*)	A suitable amount

Note: Onion juice can be substituted for scallion juice.

Method of administration: Pound the onion or scallion to extract its juice. Mix this with the powdered Tea leaves and boiling water and take.

Functions: Moistens the intestines and frees the stool

Indications: This tea is suitable for the treatment of postpartum constipation due to vacuity dryness.

Contraindications: This formula should not be taken with Rhubarb root, *i.e.*, Radix Et Rhizoma Rhei (*Da Huang*).

Honey Tea (*Mi Cha*)

Tea leaves, *i.e.*, Folium Camelliae Theae (*Cha Ye*)	3 grams
Honey (*Feng Mi*)	2ml

Method of administration: Soak these two ingredients in boiling water for 5 minutes. Each day use 1-2 packets, drinking 1 cup warm after each meal.

Functions: Moistens the intestines and frees the stools, boosts the lungs and stops coughing

Indications: This tea is suitable for the treatment of postpartum constipation, constipation in the aged, and lung dryness with a dry cough.

Corn Cob Tea (*Yu Mi Xin Cha*)

Corn cob (*Yu Mi Xin*)	30 grams
White sugar (*Bai Tang*)	Amount to taste

Method of administration: Chop the corn cob into small pieces and boil in water. Strain and add sugar to the liquid. Drink repeatedly as a tea, using 1-2 packets per day.

Functions: Boosts the qi, fortifies the spleen, and stops sweating

Indications: This tea is suitable for the treatment of postpartum vacuity sweating.

Malted Barley Weaning Tea (*Tui Na Mai Ya Cha*)

Stir-fried malted barley sprout, *i.e.,* stir-fried Fructus
    Germinatus Hordei Vulgaris (*Chao Mai Ya*)   30-60 grams

Method of administration: Boil this herb with water into a small bowl of liquid. Take 1 packet per day. Drink this warm as a tea at any time.

Functions: Stems lactation

Indications: This tea is suitable for the treatment of nursing women who want to wean their child or for lactating women who want to stop lactating for any reason.

Acute Mastitis Teas

Acute mastitis is called "breast *yong*" in TCM. Its main symptoms are breast swelling, distention, and pain or even suppuration, ulceration, and open sores. It is usually due to damage by the seven emotions or improper postpartum diet, such as eating excessively fishy, greasy, and strong-flavored foods. This results in the stomach and intestines accumulating heat with heat and toxins then congesting and stagnating in the channels and network vessels. This condition is often caused by nipple cracking or nipple malformation or inversion. Hence the milk becomes depressed and bound. The tea formulas below should be chosen based on a TCM pattern discrimination in turn based on the patient's individual signs and symptoms.

Honeysuckle & Violet Tea (*Yin Hua Di Ding Cha*)

Honeysuckle flower, *i.e.*, Flos Lonicerae Japonicae (*Jin Yin Hua*)   30 grams
Herba Violae Yedoensis Cum Radice (*Zi Hua Di Ding*)   30 grams

Method of administration: Grind the violet into a coarse powder and then boil with the honeysuckle. Drink the liquid as a tea, using 1 packet per day.

Functions: Clears heat, resolves toxins, and disperses swelling

Indications: This tea is suitable for the treatment of the initial stage of breast *yong* with fairly strong heat toxins.

Wild Chrysanthemum Flower Tea (*Ye Ju Hua Cha*)

Wild chrysanthemum flower, *i.e.*, Flos Chrysanthemi Indici
    (*Ye Ju Hua*)   15 grams

Method of administration: Steep this herb in boiling water. Use 1 packet per day. Drink the resulting liquid frequently as a tea.

Functions: Clears heat, resolves toxins, and disperses swelling

Indications: This tea is suitable for the treatment of breast *yong* at the initial stage with redness, swelling, and heat that is relatively pronounced.

Chrysanthemum & Licorice Tea (*Ju Hua Gan Cao Cha*)

Chrysanthemum flower, *i.e.*, Flos Chrysanthemi Morifolii (*Ju Hua*) 5 grams
Licorice root, *i.e.*, Radix Glycyrrhizae Uralensis (*Gan Cao*)   2.5 grams
White sugar (*Bai Tang*)   Amount to taste

180

Method of administration: Rinse the two herbs well and pour boiling water over them. Add white sugar for flavor. Drink this as a tea. Use 1 packet per day.

Functions: Clears heat and resolves toxins

Indications: This tea is suitable for the treatment of acute mastitis due to depressive heat.

Vaccaria Seed Tea (*Wang Bu Xing Cha*)

Semen Vaccariae Segetalis (*Wang Bu Liu Xing*)   15 grams

Method of administration: Boil this herb and use the liquid. Drink it as a tea, 1 packet per day.

Functions: Quickens the blood and disperses swelling, promotes lactation and scatters nodulation

Indications: This tea is suitable for the treatment of breast *yong* that is due to liver qi depression and binding and stomach heat congestion and stagnation causing the breasts to be red, swollen, and hard nodes, distention, pain, and the absence of breast milk.

Visceral Agitation Teas

The combination of mental depression, emotional vexation and derangement, abnormal laughter and weeping, and frequent yawning is called visceral agitation in Chinese medicine. It is usually due to an individual's constitution. If an individual is frequently depressed or chronically worried and anxious, their heart will become damaged. In addition, taxation and fatigue may damage the spleen. If the source of transformation of qi and blood thus becomes insufficient, then visceral yin becomes even more depleted. Visceral agitation may also be due to yin damage after an illness and postpartum hemorrhage which causes essence blood internal depletion. Yet another cause may be loss

181

of moisture and nourishment of the five viscera and/or fire transformed from excesses of the five emotions damaging internally, harassing upward and affecting the heart spirit. This then causes visceral agitation. In TCM, visceral agitation is considered a gynecological disease because yin and blood vacuity are more commonly seen in women due to their monthly menstruation and gestation, birthing, and lactation.

Licorice, Wheat & Red Dates Tea (*Gan Mai Da Zao Cha*)

Blighted wheat, *i.e.*, Semen Levis Tritici Aestivi (*Fu Xiao Mai*)	30 grams
Red dates, *i.e.*, Fructus Zizyphus Jujubae (*Da Zao*)	10 pieces
Mix-fried licorice root, *i.e.*, mix-fried Radix Glycyrrhizae Uralensis (*Zhi Gan Cao*)	6 grams

Method of administration: Boil the above ingredients, strain, and drink the liquid slowly as a tea.

Functions: Nourishes the heart and quiets the spirit, moderates sweating and harmonizes the middle

Indications: This tea is suitable for the treatment of spirit abstraction, grief damage, desire to cry, loss of self-control, frequent yawning or neurasthenia, insomnia, and night sweats due to a combination of heart and spleen vacuity with heat counterflowing upward disturbing the heart spirit and the lungs depuration and downbearing.

Codonopsis & Red Dates Tea (*Shen Zao Cha*)

Radix Codonopsitis Pilosulae (*Dang Shen*)	25 grams
Red dates, *i.e.*, Fructus Zizyphi Jujubae (*Hong Zao*)	10 grams

Note: One may also add 5 grams of tangerine peel, *i.e.*, Pericarpium Citri Reticulatae (*Chen Pi*), or replace the red dates with tangerine peel.

Method of administration: Boil the herbs with water. Take 1 packet per day and drink this warm as a tea at any time.

Functions: Supplements the spleen and harmonizes the stomach, boosts the qi and engenders liquids, regulates and harmonizes the constructive and defensive

Indications: This tea is suitable for the treatment of visceral agitation, stomach vacuity with scanty eating, post disease or postpartum spleen vacuity with loose stools, bodily emaciating, fatigue, heart palpitations, and racing heart.

Walnut & Sugar Tea (*Hu Tao Ren Tang Cha*)

Walnut, *i.e.*, Semen Juglandis Regiae (*Hu Tao Ren)*	30 grams
White sugar (*Bai Tang*)	30 grams

Method of administration: Pound the shelled walnuts into a mash. Steep along with the sugar in boiling water. Drink the resulting liquid 3 times a day.

Functions: Warms and supplements the lungs and kidneys, moistens the intestines and frees the stools

Indications: This tea is suitable for the treatment of visceral agitation primarily due to kidney vacuity.

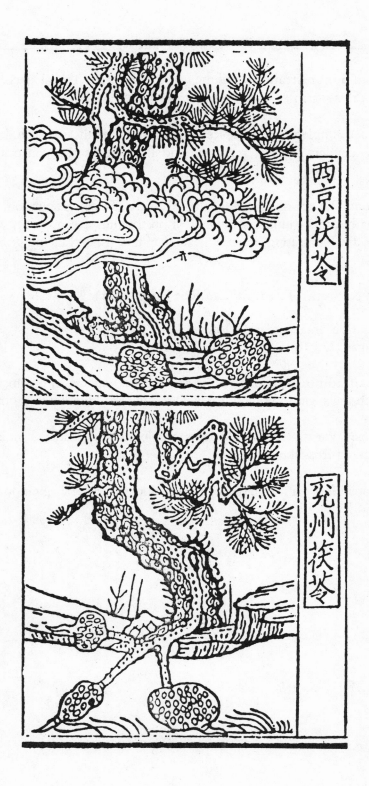

西京茯苓

兗州茯苓

11
Pediatric Diseases

Pediatric Cold & Flu Teas

Pediatric flu is a common infantile occurrence, usually caused by a contagious virus affecting the respiratory tract. Its main symptoms are aversion to cold, high fever, and sore, aching muscles and joints. In TCM, common cold and flu are usually due to invasion by wind heat or wind cold. Thus treatments focus on clearing heat and resolving toxins or dispelling wind and scattering cold.

Guanzhong Tea (*Guan Zhong Cha*)

Rhizoma Guanzhong (*Guan Zhong*)   6 grams
Green Tea, *i.e.*, Folium Camelliae Theae (*Lu Cha*)   2 grams

Method of administration: Grind these two ingredients into a coarse powder. Then steep them in boiling water for 10 minutes. An alternate method is to boil them with water. Take 1 packet per day for 5 continuous days.

Functions: Clears heat and resolves toxins, courses wind and resolves the exterior

Indications: This tea is suitable for treating pediatric flu, the common cold in any season, summerheat, and rashes all due to a wind heat exterior pattern.

Mung Bean Flu Tea (*Lu Dou Liu Gan Cha*)

Uncooked mung bean, *i.e.*, uncooked Semen Phaseoli Munginis
  (*Sheng Lu Dou*)   50 pieces

Green Tea leaves, *i.e.*, Folium Camelliae Theae (*Lu Cha Ye*)   1-3 grams
Crystal sugar (*Bing Tang*)   15 grams

Method of administration: Wash the mung beans well and pound them into pieces. Soak them with the green Tea and crystal sugar in boiling water and cover for 20 minutes. Take 1 packet per day. Drink this slowly at any time.

Functions: Clears heat, dispels wind, and resolves the exterior

Indications: This tea is suitable for the treatment of flu and has even better results for swelling and pain in the throat and heat cough all due to a wind heat exterior pattern.

Olive & Radish Tea (*Gan Lan Luo Bo Cha*)

Fresh Chinese olive, *i.e.*, fresh Fructus Canarii (*Xian Gan Lan*)   30 grams
Fresh radish, *i.e.*, uncooked Radix Raphani Sativi (*Sheng Luo Bo*) 250 grams

Method of administration: Wash the radish and chop into slices. Boil the radish slices and olives together with water. Drink the resulting liquid warm as a tea. Use 1 packet per day.

Functions: Clears heat and resolves toxins, dispels wind and resolves the exterior

Indications: This tea is suitable for the treatment of pediatric cold and flu due to a wind heat exterior pattern.

Mumps Teas

Pediatric parotitis generally refers to epidemic or infectious parotitis or what is commonly called mumps. Its clinical symptoms are pain and swelling below the jaw and in front of the ear. In TCM, this is usually due to wind warmth

186

seasonal epidemic disease contraction. It is a common contagious infantile disease, and it is important to prevent it if possible.

Two Leaves Tea (*Er Ye Cha*)

Folium Daqingye (*Da Qing Ye*)	30 grams
Dandelion, *i.e.*, Herba Cum Radice Taraxaci Mongolici (*Pu Gong Ying*)	30 grams
Herba Violae Yedoensitis Cum Radice (*Zi Hua Di Ding*)	30 grams
Green Tea leaves, *i.e.*, Folium Camelliae Theae (*Lu Cha Ye*)	9 grams

Method of administration: Boil these four ingredients. Take 1 packet per day and drink as a tea at any time.

Functions: Clears heat and resolves toxins, disperses swelling and scatters nodulation

Indications: This tea is suitable for the treatment of epidemic parotitis with parotid glands that are red, swollen, hot, and painful and accompanied by fever due to epidemic heat toxins.

Daqingye & Honeysuckle Tea (*Da Qing Ren Dong Cha*)

Folium Daqingye (*Da Qing Ye*)	30 grams
Ramus Lonicerae Japonicae (*Ren Dong Teng*)	30 grams

Method of administration: Grind the above two ingredients into a coarse powder and boil with water. Drink as a tea.

Functions: Clears, cools, and resolves toxins

Indications: This tea is suitable for the treatment of parotitis due to epidemic heat toxins.

187

Isatis & Honeysuckle Tea (*Ban Lan Yin Hua Cha*)

Radix Isatidis Seu Baphicacanthi (*Ban Lan Gen*)	30 grams
Honeysuckle flower, *i.e.*, Flos Lonicerae Japonicae (*Jin Yin Hua*)	10 grams
Field mint or peppermint, *i.e.*, Herba Menthae Haplocalycis (*Bo He*)	5 grams

Method of administration: Grind the above herbs into a coarse powder and boil with water. Drink as a tea.

Functions: Clears heat and resolves toxins

Indications: This tea is suitable for the treatment of parotitis with fever and parotid gland pain.

Whooping Cough Teas

Whooping cough or pertussis is a contagious disease typically occurring in the winter and spring caused by a respiratory tract bacterial infection (*Bordetella pertussis*). It is usually seen among children under 5 years of age. In its early stage, its symptoms are those of a typical upper respiratory tract infection. However, after 6-7 days, a paroxysmal, spastic cough occurs. This cough may be comprised of a few consecutive coughs or more then 10 coughs linked in succession and followed by inspiratory stridor like a cock crow. It is this finishing sound which gives this disease its common English name—whooping cough. This paroxysmal cough often causes vomiting and may be accompanied by facial and eyelid edema. The illness can last 4-5 weeks or more. In TCM, it is called "epidemic cough," "cormorant cough," or "hundred day cough," due to its lengthy course. Although pertussis is a nasty disease, especially in children under 1 year of age, it is rarely fatal. It is important to treat this disease properly and to prevent its transforming into pneumonia.

Loquat & Peach Seed Tea (*Pi Pa Tao Ren Cha*)

Folium Eriobotryae Japonicae (*Pi Pa Ye*)	9 grams
Peach kernel, *i.e.*, Semen Pruni Persicae (*Tao Ren*)	5 pieces

Method of administration: Clean the loquat leaves of any "down" or "hair" and then boil them together with the peach seed. Drink the resulting liquid as a tea.

Functions: Transforms phlegm, harmonizes the stomach, and downbears counterflow

Indications: This tea is suitable for the treatment of the spastic period of whooping cough with copious phlegm and vomiting.

Garlic & Crystal Sugar Tea (*Da Suan Bing Tang Cha*)

Garlic bulb, *i.e.*, Bulbus Allii Sativi (*Da Suan Tou*)	2 heads
Crystal sugar (*Bing Tang*)	Amount to taste

Method of administration: Pound the garlic into pieces and add the crystal sugar. Steep in boiling water and filter the liquid. Drink repeatedly as a tea.

Functions: Fortifies the stomach, moistens the lungs, and resolves toxins

Indications: This tea is suitable for the treatment of whooping cough.

Radish Seed Tea (*Lai Fu Cha*)

Radish seed, *i.e.*, Semen Raphani Sativi (*Lai Fu Zi*)	15 grams
White sugar (*Bai Tang*)	Amount to taste

Method of administration: Dry the radish seeds over a fire. Grind them into a fine powder. Place this powder into a teacup and pour in boiling water. White sugar can be added to taste.

Functions: Descends the qi and stabilizes dyspnea, disperses food and transforms phlegm

Indications: This tea is suitable for the treatment of whooping cough, cough, or acute and chronic bronchitis.

Peanut Tea (*Hua Sheng Cha*)

Shelled raw peanuts (*Hua Sheng*)	15 grams
Watermelon seeds, *i.e.*, Semen Citrulli Vulgaris (*Xi Gua Zi*)	15 grams
Safflower, *i.e.*, Flos Carthami Tinctorii (*Hong Hua*)	1.5 grams
Crystal sugar (*Bing Tang*)	30 grams

Note: Raw peanuts transform phlegm. Roasted peanuts engender phlegm.

Method of administration: Pound the watermelon seeds into pieces and place them and the other three ingredients into a pot. Add water, bring it to a boil, and boil for 30 minutes. Use the liquid for tea and eat the shelled peanuts. Use 1 packet per day, drunk at any time.

Functions: Diffuses the lungs and quickens the blood, transforms phlegm and settles cough

Indications: This tea is suitable for the treatment of whooping cough if the face becomes cyanotic during coughing fits.

Clematis & Crystal Sugar Tea (*Ling Xian Bing Tang Cha*)

Radix Clematidis Chinensis (*Wei Ling Xian*)	6 grams
Crystal sugar (*Bing Tang*)	50 grams

Method of administration: Boil these two ingredients together. Drink the resulting liquid as a tea.

Functions: Disperses phlegm and stops cough

190

Indications: This tea is suitable for the treatment of whooping cough during the spastic period with paroxysmal cough and phlegm binding in the throat.

Pediatric Measles Teas

Measles is one of the four major diseases that affect children. It is both acute and contagious. It can occur at any time of the year but usually strikes during the winter and spring. Clinically, its main symptoms are fever, cough, a clear runny nose, and then the eruption of the measles rash all over the body. Measles in TCM is believed to be due to yang toxins. Out-thrusting these toxins leads to a favorable resolution. Thus, the treatment for measles in its initial stage focuses on promoting the out-thrusting or eruption of the measles. After the measles have been out-thrust, treatment focuses on clearing heat and resolving toxins. During the later or last stage, treatment focuses on boosting the qi and nourishing yin. It is contraindicated to use any warm, acid, downward attacking (*i.e.*, precipitating or purging), very bitter and cold medicinals. In order to apply the correct formula, treatment should be based on the different stages of the disease and the patient's particular pattern.

Children's Measles Tea (*Xiao Er Ma Zhen Cha*)

Fresh shepherd's purse, *i.e.*, fresh Herba Capsellae Bursa-pastoris (*Xian Ji Cai*)	100 grams
Rhizoma Imperatae Cylindricae (*Bai Mao Gen*)	50 grams

Method of administration: Wash the above two herbs well. Place them in a pot, add 500ml of water, and boil for 10-15 minutes. Use 1 packet per day and drink the resulting liquid in 2 doses.

Functions: Harmonizes the spleen and disinhibits water, clears heat and resolves toxins

Indications: This tea is suitable for the treatment of pediatric measles fire exuberance and also to prevent the contraction of epidemic measles.

191

Children's Out-thrusting the Rash Tea (*Xiao Er Tou Zhen Cha*)

Sugarcane (*Gan Zhe*)   100 grams
Water chestnut (*Bi Qi*)   100 grams
Carrot (*Hu Luo Bo*)   100 grams

Method of administration: Wash these three ingredients well and cut them into small cubes. Place in a pot and add 500ml of water. Boil until 250ml of liquid is left. Drink the resulting liquid as a tea.

Functions: Clears heats and nourishes yin, engenders fluids and moistens dryness

Indications: This tea is suitable for the treatment of childhood measles.

Bupleurum & Phragmites Tea (*Chai Lu Cha*)

Radix Bupleuri (*Chai Hu*)   6 grams
Rhizoma Phragmitis Communis (*Lu Gen*)   15 grams

Method of administration: Grind these two herbs into a coarse powder. Steep in boiling water. Drink this frequently as a tea.

Functions: Clears heat and courses the exterior

Indications: This tea is suitable for the treatment or the prevention of measles during an epidemic period.

Beet & Water Chestnut Tea (*Hong Luo Bo Bi Qi Cha*)

Beet (*Hong Luo Bo*)   250-400 grams
Water chestnut (*Bi Qi*)   250-400 grams

Method of administration: Wash the above two ingredients well and boil with water. Drink the resulting liquid warm as a tea at any time. Take 1 packet per day.

Functions: Clears heat and resolves toxins, nourishes yin and engenders fluids

Indications: This tea is suitable for the treatment of childhood measles and summerheat.

Carrot & Coriander Tea (*Luo Bo Xiang Cai Cha*)

Carrot (*Hu Luo Bo*)	120 grams
Coriander (*Xiang Cai*)	100 grams
Water chestnut (*Bi Qi*)	60 grams

Method of administration: Wash the above three ingredients well and boil with water. Use 1 packet per day. Drink the resulting liquid warm at any time.

Functions: Clears heat and resolves toxins, dispels wind and out-thrusts the rash

Indications: This tea is suitable for the treatment of pediatric measles heat toxins. It can also enable rapid eruption of the measles rash, thus decreasing the child's suffering since the resolution of the disease goes along with the complete and successful eruption of the rash.

Pediatric Rubella Teas

Rubella or so-called German measles is a relatively mild contagious disease accompanied by the eruption of a rash. It occurs usually among children 1-5 years old and often occurs between the winter and spring. Its main clinical manifestation is the appearance of small, light red papules on the skin either locally or all over the body. These papules appear and disappear fairly quickly and leave no scars or marks behind. In TCM, this condition is usually due to externally contracted wind heat that is depressed in the flesh and muscle exterior. It may also be due to blood vacuity engendering wind and the skin lacking nourishment. Treatment should focus on clearing heat and dispelling wind, resolving toxins and dissipating papules, or nourishing the blood and dispelling wind.

Forsythia & Burdock Tea (*Lian Bang Cha*)

Forsythia fruit, *i.e.*, Fructus Forsythiae Suspensae (*Lian Qiao*)	6 grams
Burdock seed, *i.e.*, Fructus Arctii Lappae (*Niu Bang Zi*)	5 grams
Green Tea, *i.e.*, Folium Camelliae Theae (*Lu Cha*)	1 gram

Method of administration: Grind these three ingredients into a powder and steep this powder in boiling water. An alternate method is to boil these ingredients for a brief time. Use 1 packet per day. Drink the resulting liquid warm as a tea at any time.

Functions: Dissipates heat and dispels wind, diffuses the lungs and out-thrusts the rash

Indications: This tea is suitable for the treatment of rubella and measles manifesting as a wind heat pattern.

Dissipate the Rash Tea (*San Zhen Cha*)

Uncooked Radix Rehmanniae (*Sheng Di*)	90 grams
Rhizoma Atractylodis (*Cang Zhu*)	30 grams
Tea leaves, *i.e.*, Folium Camelliae Theae (*Cha Ye*)	10 grams

If under 5 years old:

Uncooked Radix Rehmanniae (*Sheng Di*)	9 grams
Rhizoma Atractylodis (*Cang Zhu*)	3-6 grams
Tea leaves, *i.e.*, Folium Camelliae Theae (*Cha Ye*)	1-3 grams

Method of administration: Boil the first two herbs in water and then use the liquid to make the Tea. Take 1 packet per day. Drink the liquid slowly until a sweat appears all over the body. This tea may be taken at any time of day.

Functions: Nourishes the blood, dispels wind, and dissipates the rash

Indications: This tea is suitable for the treatment of either rubella or urticaria due to a combination of dampness and yin vacuity heat.

Contraindications: After taking this formula and sweating, it is contraindicated to be exposed to drafts or cold so as to avoid wind damage and contraction of cold.

Honeysuckle & Cicada Tea (*Yin Chan Cha*)

Honeysuckle flower, *i.e.*, Flos Lonicerae Japonicae (*Jin Yin Hua*)	3-6 grams
Periostracum Cicadae (*Chan Tui*)	1-3 grams
Green Tea, *i.e.*, Folium Camelliae Theae (*Lu Cha*)	1 gram
Licorice root, *i.e.*, Radix Glycyrrhizae Uralensis (*Gan Cao*)	1 gram

Method of administration: Grind the four ingredients into a coarse powder and steep in boiling water for 10 minutes. An alternate method is to boil the above ingredients with water and drink this as a tea. Use 1 packet per day.

Functions: Clears heat and resolves toxins, dispels wind and dissipates the rash

Indications: This tea is suitable for the treatment of rubella, urticaria, and measles when exhibiting a wind heat pattern.

Contraindications: Eating of raw, cold foods and exposure to cold are contraindicated.

Pediatric Chickenpox Teas

Chickenpox or varicella is an acute disease caused by the *Varicella-Zoster* virus infection. It is highly contagious and may be epidemic. Its main characteristics are fever and skin and mucous membrane eruptions that pass through several stages: macule to papule to vesicle to crusts. It usually affects children from 1-6 years old. In TCM, this disease is believed to be due to externally contracted seasonal evil toxins, internal dampness, and smoldering of depressed heat. It may be prevented and treated by the following herbal tea formulas according to the individual's pattern of disharmony.

Chinese Olive & Phragmites Tea (*Qing Guo Lu Gen Cha*)

Chinese olive, *i.e.*, Fructus Canarii (*Qing Guo*)	30 grams
Rhizoma Phragmitis Communis (*Lu Gen*)	60 grams

Method of administration: Pound the olives into pieces and cut the phragmites into pieces. Boil these together with water and drink the resulting liquid as a tea.

Functions: Clears heat and resolves toxins, engenders fluids and disinhibits the throat

Indications: This tea is suitable for the treatment of chickenpox during its initial stage with fever and a red, painful throat or, in other words, when it exhibits a wind heat exterior pattern.

Phragmites & Chrysanthemum Tea (*Lu Ju Cha*)

Rhizoma Phragmitis Communis (*Lu Gen*)	60 grams
Wild chrysanthemum flower, *i.e.*, Flos Chrysanthemi Indici (*Ye Ju Hua*)	10 grams

Method of administration: Cut the phragmites into pieces and then boil these pieces and the chrysanthemum flowers with water. Drink the liquid as a tea.

Functions: Clears heat and resolves toxins, engenders fluids and stops thirst

Indications: This tea is suitable for the treatment of chickenpox manifesting as a pattern of heat toxins.

Pediatric Stagnant Food Teas

Accumulation and stagnation refers to a type of chronic pediatric gastro-intestinal disease which is due to food stagnation that collects and gathers without being transformed. This results in qi stagnation and lack of movement of the digestate. In TCM, accumulation and stagnation are closely related to milk damage and food damage. Milk and food damage refer to damage due to over-feeding of milk and/or food which then cannot be digested properly by the infant's inherently weak spleen and stomach. If this condition becomes chronic, it develops from food stagnation into accumulation. If accumulation is not treated in time, it may then transform into pediatric *gan* or malnutrition due to digestive disturbance or intestinal parasites. Although pediatric *gan* is seldom seen in the West, pediatric food stagnation is the root of many of the most common pediatric complaints, such as colic, earache, nasal congestion, and coughs. Therefore, the treatment of pediatric food stagnation in its early stages is important in order to prevent other pediatric conditions.

Transform Accumulation Tea (*Hua Ji Cha*)

Hawthorn fruit, *i.e.*, Fructus Crataegi (*Shan Zha*)	15 grams
Malted barley, *i.e.*, Fructus Germinatus Hordei Vulgaris (*Mai Ya*)	10 grams
Radish seed, *i.e.*, Semen Raphani Sativi (*Lai Fu Zi*)	8 grams
Rhubarb root, *i.e.*, Radix Et Rhizoma Rhei (*Da Huang*)	2 grams

Method of administration: Place the above four ingredients in a cup and steep in boiling water for a few moments. Drink 1 packet per day as a tea.

Functions: Disperses food and transforms accumulation

Indications: This tea is suitable for the treatment of undigested and accumulated food with a poor appetite, bad breath, and possible colic in infants.

Rice Tea (*Mi Cha*)

Semen Oryzae Sativae (*Da Mi*)	100 grams
Tea leaves, *i.e.*, Folium Camelliae Theae (*Cha Ye*)	6 grams

Method of administration: Rinse the rice well and place in a pot with a suitable amount of water. Soak the Tea leaves in boiling water for 6 minutes. Pour the Tea water into the rice and make a rice gruel. Take this once a day, eating it warm.

Functions: Fortifies the spleen, harmonizes the stomach, and disperses accumulation

Indications: This tea is suitable for the treatment of pediatric indigestion due to food stagnation.

Agastaches & Eupatorium Tea (*Huo Pei Cha*)

Herba Agastachis Seu Pogostemi (*Huo Xiang*)	3 grams
Herba Eupatorii Fortunei (*Pei Lan*)	6 grams
Field mint or peppermint, *i.e.*, Herba Menthae Haplocalycis (*Bo He*)	4.5 grams
Cardamon, *i.e.*, Fructus Cardamomi (*Bai Dou Kou*)	1.5 grams

Method of administration: Grind the above four ingredients into a coarse powder and steep in boiling water. Cover for 10 minutes and drink as a tea. Use 1 packet per day.

Functions: Transforms dampness, disperses stagnation, and arouses the stomach

Indications: This tea is suitable for the treatment of the excessive eating of fatty and greasy foods, indigestion, torpid intake, decreased food intake, a sticky, greasy sensation with no taste in the mouth, bad breath, and a sour, foul mouth upon waking.

Three Fresh (Ingredients) Disperse Food Tea (*San Xian Xiao Shi Cha*)

Fresh hawthorn fruit, *i.e.*, fresh Fructus Crataegi (*Xian Shan Zha*) 20 grams
Fresh white radish, *i.e.*, Radix Raphani Sativi (*Xian Bai Luo Bo*)   30 grams
Fresh tangerine peel, *i.e.*, fresh Pericarpium Citri Reticulatae
   (*Xian Ju Pi*)   5 grams
Crystal sugar (*Bing Tang*)   Amount to taste

Method of administration: Rinse the hawthorn fruit, white radish, and tangerine peel well. Pat the hawthorn fruit into pieces, cut the white radish into small cubes, and tear the tangerine peel into pieces. Place all into a pot, add 500ml of water, and boil for 10-15 minutes. Then add the crystal sugar to taste. Use the liquid and drink it as a tea.

Functions: Disperses food and transforms accumulation

Indications: This tea is suitable for the treatment of children's milk food collection and stagnation as well as pediatric *gan* accumulation.

Carrot Tea (*Hu Luo Bo Cha*)

Carrot (*Hu Luo Bo*)   250 grams
Brown sugar (*Hong Tang*)   Amount to taste

Method of administration: Boil the carrot with water. Then add a little brown sugar. Drink the resulting liquid as a tea repeatedly.

Functions: Moves the qi and disperses food

Indications: This tea is suitable for the treatment of pediatric accumulation and stagnation, abdominal distention, untransformed accumulated food, constant vomiting and diarrhea, and constant crying and fussiness all due to food stagnation.

Pediatric Diarrhea Teas

Pediatric diarrhea is a common gastrointestinal tract disturbance. Clinically, its main characteristics are increased frequency of defecation, watery, loose stools, stools like egg flower water, or stools mixed with undigested food. In China, pediatric diarrhea usually occurs in autumn, especially in children under 2 years of age. The younger the child is, the more changeable is the condition. When severe, fluids can be lost rapidly and vacuity desertion will occur. If the diarrhea lingers or occurs repeatedly, malnutrition and *gan* disease may develop. In TCM, pediatric diarrhea is divided into damp heat diarrhea, food damage diarrhea, and spleen vacuity diarrhea.

Pediatric Diarrhea Green Tea (*Ying Er Xie Xie Lu Cha*)

Green Tea from Yunnan, *i.e.*, Yunnan Folium Camelliae Theae
   (*Yun Nan Lu Cha*)   1 gram

Method of administration: Grind the Tea into a very fine powder. For simple infantile diarrhea, use 1 gram of Tea powder 3 times per day. Stir this into warm water or mother's milk. Administer it continuously for 1-4 days.

Functions: Clears heat, disperses food, and stops diarrhea

Indications: This tea is suitable for the treatment of infantile diarrhea due to heat transformed from stagnant food.

200

Malted Barley Tea (*Mai Cha*)

Stir-fried malted barley, *i.e.*, stir-fried Fructus Germinatus Hordei Vulgaris (*Chao Mai Ya*)	30 grams
Tea leaves stir-fried till scorched, *i.e.*, stir-fried till scorched Folium Camelliae Theae (*Chao Jiao Cha Ye*)	8 grams

Method of administration: Soak these two ingredients in boiling water. Take the resulting liquid as a tea.

Functions: Disperses food and stops diarrhea

Indications: This tea is suitable for the treatment of infantile food damage diarrhea, watery, loose stools mixed with undigested food and/or curdled milk which are sour and foul smelling, burping, and lack of appetite.

Mugwort & Ginger Tea (*Ai Ye Jiang Cha*)

Mugwort, *i.e.*, Folium Artemisiae Argyii (*Ai Ye*)	6 grams
Uncooked ginger, *i.e.*, uncooked Rhizoma Zingiberis (*Sheng Jiang*)	2 slices

Method of administration: Boil these two ingredients and strain off the liquid. Take this as a tea.

Functions: Warms the middle and scatters cold

Indications: This tea is suitable for the treatment of cold diarrhea. When cold pathogens settle in the intestines and stomach, the intestines rumble with abdominal pain, there is watery diarrhea, and the infant cries and is uncomfortable. After burping, the crying stops.

Umeboshi & Terminalia Stop Diarrhea Tea (*Wu He Zhi Xie Cha*)

Umeboshi, *i.e.*, Fructus Pruni Mume (*Wu Mei*)	2 grams
Fructus Terminaliae Chebulae (*He Zi*)	3 grams

201

Method of administration: Rinse these two ingredients well and then steep them in boiling water in a teacup. Use 1 packet per day. Take the resulting liquid warm, 5-6 doses per day.

Functions: Astringes the intestines and stops diarrhea

Indications: This tea is suitable for the treatment of chronic, incessant infantile diarrhea. In this case, enduring diarrhea has damaged the kidney qi's securing and astringing function, remembering that the kidneys govern the anus and urethra and also govern opening and closing.

Contraindications: This tea is not suitable for infantile diarrhea of only a few days duration. Otherwise, evil qi may be retained to smolder and fume internally.

Pediatric Enuresis Teas

Nocturnal enuresis is also called bed-wetting and refers to urinating uncontrollably during sleep. It often occurs in young children, due to children's inherently immature kidneys. In TCM, it is, therefore, usually due to kidney qi insufficiency and vacuity cold of the lower origin. It may also be due to bodily weakness after disease resulting in lung and spleen qi vacuity not containing. In some cases, it may be due to damp heat in turn caused by faulty diet. The aforementioned patterns do not include enuresis due to organic pathology.

Alpinia Oxyphylla Draw Back the Urine Tea (*Yi Zhi Suo Niao Cha*)

Black cardamon, *i.e.*, Fructus Alpiniae Oxyphyllae (*Yi Zhi Ren*)	6 grams
Fructus Rosae Laevigatae (*Jin Ying Zi*)	6 grams
Radix Linderae Strychnifoliae (*Wu Yao*)	5 grams

Method of administration: Boil these three ingredients in 1 bowl of water until half a bowl is left. Take 1 packet per day, drunk slowly as a tea.

Functions: Banks the origin and supplements the kidneys, dispels cold and stops urination

Indications: This tea is suitable for the treatment of enuresis due to kidney vacuity with copious, clear, and long urination.

Polygonatum Tea (*Yu Zhu Cha*)

Solomon's seal, *i.e.*, Rhizoma Polygonati Odorati (*Yu Zhu*)   50 grams

Method of administration: Rinse the herb well and boil with water. Drink as a tea.

Functions: Supplements yin and boosts the kidneys

Indications: This tea is suitable for the treatment of childhood enuresis due to a weak constitution, insecure kidney qi with copious urine, and nocturnal enuresis.

Fortify the Child Tea (*Jian Er Cha*)

Red dates, *i.e.*, Fructus Zizyphi Jujubae (*Da Zao*)	50 grams
Tea leaves, *i.e.*, Folium Camelliae Theae (*Cha Ye*)	3 grams
White sugar (*Bai Tang*)	Amount to taste

Method of administration: Steep the Tea leaves in boiling water and save the Tea water for use. Cook the dates completely, add the white sugar and the Tea water, stir evenly, and drink.

Functions: Fortifies the spleen and harmonizes the stomach

Indications: This tea is suitable for the treatment of childhood enuresis due to spleen qi vacuity.

203

Infantile Night-crying Teas

Night-crying refers to infants under 3 months who cry at night without apparent cause. This is what we in the West call pediatric colic. As the sun goes down, the baby begins to cry and fuss. Typically, they pump their knees to their chest in an effort to expel gas. If they succeed in passing gas, their crying stops temporarily. Otherwise, the child demands to be carried and rocked constantly. This condition is divided into cold and hot patterns and commonly is transformed from food stagnation due to unregulated feeding.

Juncus Tea (*Deng Xin Cao Cha*)

Medulla Junci Effusi (*Deng Xin Cao*)	2 grams
Herba Lophatheri Gracilis (*Dan Zhu Ye*)	10 pieces

Method of administration: Steep these two ingredients in boiling water. Administer to the infant as a tea.

Functions: Clears the heart and eliminates vexation

Indications: This tea is suitable for the treatment of infantile vexation of the heart and night-crying due to heat. When the baby cries, their face gets red and their hands and feet are hot or warm to the touch.

Perilla & Coptis Tea (*Su Lian Cha*)

Perilla leaf, *i.e.*, Folium Perillae Frutescentis (*Zi Su Ye*)	3 grams
Rhizoma Coptidis Chinensis (*Huang Lian*)	1 gram

Method of administration: Steep the above two herbs in boiling water. Administer to the infant as a tea.

Functions: Rectifies the qi and clears heat

Indications: This tea is suitable for the treatment of night crying due to heat in turn transformed from food stagnation.

Pediatric Drooling Teas

Pediatric drooling refers to drooling constantly from the corner of the mouth. Clinically in TCM, it is often divided into two types: cold and hot. Both are caused by spleen vacuity not containing.

Ginger, Sugar & Massa Medica Fermentata Tea
(*Jiang Tang Shen Qu Cha*)

Uncooked ginger, *i.e.*, uncooked Rhizoma Zingiberis (*Sheng Jiang*)   2 slices
Massa Medica Fermentata (*Shen Qu*)   ½ piece
White sugar (*Bai Tang*)   Amount to taste

Method of administration: Place these three ingredients in a pot, add some water, and cook slightly. Administer the resulting liquid as a tea.

Functions: Fortifies the spleen, warms the middle, and stops drooling

Indications: This tea is suitable for the treatment of pediatric drooling.

Red Date, Tangerine Peel & Lophatherum Tea
(*Da Zao Chen Pi Zhu Ye Cha*)

Red dates, *i.e.*, Fructus Zizyphi Jujubae (*Da Zao*)   5 pieces
Tangerine peel, *i.e.*, Pericarpium Citri Reticulatae (*Chen Pi*)   5 grams
Herba Lophatheri Gracilis (*Dan Zhu Ye*)   7 grams

Method of administration: Boil the above three herbs with water. Take 1 packet twice a day for 3-5 days continuously.

Functions: Fortifies the spleen, boosts the qi, and stops drooling

Indications: This tea is suitable for the treatment of pediatric drooling due to spleen qi vacuity.

12
Diseases of the Eyes, Ears, Nose, Throat & Head

Acute Conjunctivitis Teas

Acute conjunctivitis is commonly called "red eyes" or "fire eyes" in Chinese and is a common contagious eye disease. In light cases, the symptoms are hypereremia of the conjunctiva, itchy eyes, and a sensation of a foreign object and burning heat in the eye. In severe cases, the symptoms are swelling of the eyelid and hemorrhage or corneal infiltration and ulceration.

Chrysanthemum & Dragon Well Tea (*Ju Hua Long Jing Cha*)

Chrysanthemum flower, *i.e.*, Flos Chrysanthemi Morifolii (*Ju Hua*) 10 grams
Dragon Well Tea, *i.e.*, Dragon Well Folium Camelliae Theae
    (*Long Jing Cha*) 3 grams

Note: Dragon Well Tea is grown in Hangzhou, Zhejiang province in the vicinity of the Dragon Well and hence its name. It is considered one of the best varietal teas of China.

Method of administration: Steep these two ingredients in boiling water for 5-10 minutes. Use 1 packet per day, drunk as a tea at any time.

Functions: Courses wind, clears heat, and brightens the eyes

Indications: This tea is suitable for the treatment of liver fire exuberance that causes reddening of the eyes, shying away from brightness, photophobia, and acute conjunctivitis due to wind heat.

Contraindications: Hot, acrid, spicy foods, greasy foods, and alcohol are forbidden to patients with the above heat conditions.

Scutellaria Tea (*Huang Qin Cha*)

Radix Scutellariae Baicalensis (*Huang Qin*)   15 grams

Method of administration: Grind this herb into a coarse powder and steep in boiling water. Drink this as a tea.

Functions: Clears heat, drains fire, and brightens the eyes

Indications: This tea is suitable for the treatment of upper burner lung fire exuberance or depressed heat causing acute conjunctivitis.

Buddleia Tea (*Mi Meng Hua Cha*)

Flos Buddleiae Officinalis (*Mi Meng Hua*)   5 grams
Green Tea, *i.e.*, Folium Camelliae Theae (*Lu Cha*)   1 gram
Honey sugar (*Mi Tang*)   25 grams

Method of administration: Boil the buddleia flower and the green Tea in 350ml of water for 3 minutes. Filter it through gauze and add the honey sugar to the liquid. Bring back to a boil and then drink the resulting liquid. Take 1 packet per day. Drink this frequently as a tea.

Functions: Clears the liver and drains heat, brightens the eyes and abates eye-screen

Indications: This tea is suitable for the treatment of shying away from brightness and fearing light, excessive exudation from the eyes, excessive tearing, eye-clouding, and eye-screen.

Cassia & Chrysanthemum Flower Tea (*Jue Ming Ju Hua Cha*)

Ground Semen Cassiae Torae (*Dao Sui Jue Ming Zi*)   10 grams
Chrysanthemum flower, *i.e.*, Flos Chrysanthemi Morifolii (*Ju Hua*) 3 grams
Sliced hawthorn fruit, *i.e.,* Fructus Crataegi (*Shan Zha Pian*)   15 grams

Method of administration: Place these three ingredients in a thermos, steep in boiling water, and cover for 30 minutes. Take 1 packet per day, drunk as a tea.

Functions: Clears the liver and brightens the eyes, disinhibits the urine and frees the stools

Indications: This tea is suitable for the treatment of red eye with swelling pain, headache, dizziness, cloudy, dry, and astringent eyes, and decreased eyesight. It is also suitable for hypertension with clouded and red eyes, dry, bound stools, ascites due to cirrhosis, and habitual constipation.

Clear the Liver & Brighten the Eyes Tea (*Qing Gan Ming Mu Cha*)

Semen Cassiae Torae (*Jue Ming Zi*)   25 grams
Motherwort seed , *i.e.*, Semen Leonuri Heterophylli *Chong Wei Zi*) 10 grams

Method of administration: Stir-fry the above two herbs over a gentle fire. Then press them into pieces. Place these into a pot, boil for 20 minutes, and use the liquid. Drink this as a tea, 1 packet per day.

Functions: Dispels wind and dissipates heat, clears the liver and brightens the eyes

Indications: This tea is suitable for the treatment or prevention of acute conjunctivitis in the summertime.

Blepharitis Teas

Blepharitis refers to a subacute or chronic inflammation of the margin of the eyelids, eyelash hair follicles, and local sebaceous glands. Its main symptoms are redness of the skin, infiltration, and erosion possibly accompanied by sharp itching, the sensation of a foreign object in the eyes, or a burning sensation. It may albo be due to allergies, exposure to smoke, dust, chemicals, or a bacterial infection (usually *Staphylococcus*).

Disperse Inflammation Eye Wash Tea (*Xiao Yan Xi Yan Cha*)

Good quality Green Tea, *i.e.*, Folium Camelliae Theae (*Lu Cha*)   25 grams

Method of administration: Boil the tea in 1,500-2,000ml of water until 1,000ml of liquid is left. Use this liquid after its temperature has become temperate. Use 1 packet per day. Use a piece of clean towel or gauze to wet and wash the diseased eye. Wash it 3-4 times a day.

Functions: Disperses inflammation and brightens the eyes

Indications: This tea is suitable for the treatment of blepharitis or acute conjunctivitis.

Erosion of the Eye External Wash Tea (*Lan Yan Wai Xi Cha*)

Radix Gentianae Scabrae (*Long Dan Cao*)   9 grams
Tea leaves, *i.e.*, Folium Camelliae Theae (*Cha Ye*)   9 grams
Alumen (*Bai Fan)*   3 grams
Salt (*Yan*)   3 grams
Safflower, *i.e.*, Flos Carthami Tinctorii (*Hong Hua*)   3 grams
Licorice root, *i.e.*, Radix Glycyrrhizae Uralensis (*Gan Cao*) 3 grams
Prepared Alumen (*Ku Fan)*   6 grams
Radix Ledebouriellae Divaricatae (*Fang Feng*)   6 grams
Mulberry leaf, *i.e.*, Folium Mori Albi (*Sang Ye*)   6 grams
Uncooked apricot kernel, *i.e.*, uncooked Semen Pruni Armeniacae
    (*Sheng Xing Ren*)   7 pieces

210

Chrysanthemum flower, *i.e.*, Flos Chrysanthemi Morifolii (*Ju Hua*)   10 grams

Method of administration: Boil the above herbs together with water. Use the liquid to wash the eye externally. Use 1 packet per day. Fumigate and wash the eye a few times a day with this liquid.

Functions: Clears heat and resolves toxins, dispels and transforms dampness

Indications: This tea is suitable for the treatment of wind fire erosion of the eye with itching.

Contraindications: Use as an external eye wash only. *Do not drink.*

Decreased Visual Acuity Teas

Hypopsia or decreased visual acuity refers to the gradual decrease of eyesight. In TCM, this is due to liver and kidney depletion and vacuity among young, middle-aged, and elderly people. This condition includes nearsightedness (myopia) and night blindness (nyctalopia).

Lycium & Chrysanthemum Tea (*Qi Ju Cha*)

Fructus Lycii Chinensis (*Gou Qi Zi*)   10 grams
White chrysanthemum flower, *i.e.*, Flos Chrysanthemi Morifolii
    (*Bai Ju Hua*)   10 grams
Good quality Green Tea, *i.e.*, Folium Camelliae Theae (*Lu Cha*)   3 grams

Method of administration: Steep these three ingredients in boiling water for 10 minutes and then drink. Use 1 packet per day. This may be taken repeatedly at any time.

Functions: Nourishes the liver and enriches the kidneys, courses wind and brightens the eyes

Indications: This tea is suitable for the treatment of diminished visual acuity, vertigo, night blindness, and nearsightedness in the young.

Lycium Soak Tea (*Gou Qi Pao Cha*)

Fructus Lycii Chinensis (*Gou Qi Zi*)   20 grams

Method of administration: Steep this herb in boiling water. Use 1 packet per day. Drink this repeatedly.

Functions: Supplements the kidneys and boosts the essence, nourishes the liver and brightens the eyes

Indications: This tea is suitable for the treatment of diminished visual acuity, shying away from brightness, and night blindness in the aged. It can also be used for cataracts in the elderly and vitreous opacity.

Nasal Sinusitis Teas

Sinusitis is divided into acute and chronic types. The main symptoms of acute sinusitis are nasal congestion, runny, purulent nasal mucous, and head distention or headache. Accompanying symptoms may include fever, fear of cold, poor appetite, and general malaise. This is a common nasal condition and is a complication of acute rhinitis. Chronic systemic disease, malnutrition, contraction of cold, catching a chill, habitual drinking of alcohol and smoking of tobacco can all be contributing factors. The common pathogenic bacteria are *Streptococcus*, *Staphylococcus*, *Pneumococcus*, and *Influenza bacillus*. Chronic sinusitis is usually due to a worsening of acute nasal sinusitis. Its main symptoms are nasal congestion, a purulent, fishy or foul smelling secretion from either one or both nostrils, dizziness, headache, decreased sense of smell, difficulty concentrating, and impaired memory. In TCM, nasal sinusitis belongs to the category of "deep source nasal congestion." Its acute form is mostly due to external invasion of wind heat, while its chronic form is mostly due to depressive heat in the lungs, liver, and stomach with spleen vacuity and dampness.

212

Szechuan Phellodendron Tea (*Chuan Huang Bai Cha*)

Cortex Phellodendri (*Huang Bai*)	6 grams
Dragon Well Tea, *i.e.*, Dragon Well Folium Camelliae Theae (*Long Jing Cha*)	30 grams

Method of administration: Grind the above two ingredients into a powder and store. When needed, pick up a small amount and sniff it into the nose on both sides. This snuff may be used 5-6 times each day.

Functions: Clears heat and drains fire, resolves toxins and expels pus

Indications: This tea is suitable for the treatment of deep source nasal congestion and nasal congestion with purulent secretion that has a fishy, foul smell in the nasal cavity.

Xanthium Tea (*Cang Er Zi Cha*)

Fructus Xanthii (*Cang Er Zi*)	12 grams
Flos Magnoliae Liliflorae (*Xin Yi*)	6 grams
Radix Angelicae Dahuricae (*Bai Zhi*)	6 grams
Field mint or peppermint, *i.e.*, Herba Menthae Haplocalycis (*Bo He*)	4.5 grams
Scallion, *i.e.*, Herba Allii Fistulosi (*Cong Bai*)	3 stalks
Tea leaves, *i.e.*, Folium Camelliae Theae (*Cha Ye*)	2 grams

Method of administration: Grind these six ingredients into powder and steep in boiling water for 10 minutes. Use 1 packet per day. Drink this warm repeatedly at any time.

Functions: Promotes sweating and frees the portals, dissipates wind and dispels dampness

Indications: This tea is suitable for treating the symptoms of acute rhinitis, nasal sinusitis, and accessory nasal sinusitis.

Magnoliae Flower Tea (*Xin Yi Cha*)

Flos Magnoliae Liliflorae (*Xin Yi*)	2 grams
Perilla leaf, *i.e.*, Folium Perillae Frutescentis (*Zi Su Ye*)	6 grams

Method of administration: Grind the above two ingredients into a coarse powder, wrap in gauze, and soak with boiled water. Drink this as a tea. Take 1 packet per day.

Functions: Dissipates wind and cold and frees the nasal portals

Indications: This tea is suitable for the symptomatic treatment of acute and chronic rhinitis as well as allergic rhinitis.

Nosebleed Teas

Nosebleed or epistaxis is a common condition. Usually the bleeding is only from one side and originates from the anterior, lower part of the nasal septum. There are many causes for bleeding from the nose, such as external injury, dryness of the nasal mucous, ulceration, inflammation of the nasal cavity, acute febrile infectious disease, vitamin deficiency, hypertension, or various blood diseases. Long-term, repeated nosebleeds can cause secondary anemia.

Imperata Tea (*Bai Mao Gen Cha*)

Rhizoma Imperatae Cylindricae (*Bai Mao Gen*)	15 grams

Method of administration: Boil this herb with water and drink the resulting tea.

Functions: Courses wind and stops bleeding

Indications: This tea is suitable for the treatment of nosebleed that is due to wind heat harassing above causing recurrent nosebleed.

Lycium Root Bark Tea (*Di Gu Pi Cha*)

Cortex Radicis Lycii Chinensis (*Di Gu Pi*)   20 grams

Method of administration: Grind this herb into a coarse powder and steep in boiling water. Use 1 packet per day. Drink this as a tea.

Functions: Clears heat and cools the blood

Indications: This tea is suitable for the treatment of nosebleeds and gingival bleeding due to blood heat.

Otitis Media Tea

Otitis media refers to an acute inflammation of the middle ear. It is common among children. Its main symptoms are sudden ear pain, fever, and decreased hearing. If this is not treated in a timely and proper manner, this can develop into a chronic, recurring condition. If the eardrum ruptures, which it usually does not, then there will be pus suppurating from the auditory meatus or opening of the ear.

Phellodendron & Xanthium Tea (*Huang Bai Cang Er Cha*)

Cortex Phellodendri (*Huang Bai*)   9 grams
Fructus Xanthii (*Cang Er Zi*)   10 grams
Green Tea, *i.e.*, Folium Camelliae Theae (*Lu Cha*)   3 grams

Method of administration: Grind the above three ingredients into powder and steep in boiling water for 10 minutes. These ingredients may also be boiled into a tea. Use 1 packet per day taken in 2 divided doses.

Functions: Clears heat and transforms dampness, expels pus and resolves toxins, frees the portal of the ear

215

Indications: This tea is suitable for the treatment of otitis media due to heat.

Tongue & Mouth Sores Teas

Sores on the tongue and in the mouth refer to white ulcerous blisters that occur in the mouth, on the insides of the cheeks, or on the edges of the lips or tongue. They are usually accompanied by redness, swelling, and pain. In English, these are usually called canker sores. In Chinese, they are called "oral putrescence" and "oral break." Clinically, they can be categorized as either replete or vacuity conditions. Replete conditions are usually due to damage in the oral cavity together with evil toxins or spleen and stomach heat accumulation. The repletion type occurs quickly and is easy to cure. The vacuity condition is usually due to vacuity fire flaming upward. It develops slowly, is more difficult to cure, and usually occurs repeatedly.

Terra Flava Usta & Lophatherum Tea (*Zhao Xin Tu Zhu Ye Cha*)

Terra Flava Usta (*Fu Long Gan*)	Equal amount
Herba Lophatheri Gracilis (*Dan Zhu Ye*)	Equal amount

Method of administration: First, boil the terra flava usta and wait until it settles. Then use the cleared liquid and lophatherum and boil again. Drink the resulting liquid as a tea.

Functions: Warms the middle and dries dampness, disinhibits below and clears above

Indications: This tea is suitable for the treatment of ulcerative stomatitis and stomatitis due to heart/ spleen yin fluid insufficiency and vacuity fire with frenetic movement flaming upward to the mouth and tongue.

Lophatherum Leaf Tea (*Dan Zhu Ye Cha*)

Herba Lophatheri Gracilis (*Dan Zhu Ye*)	15 grams

Method of administration: Cut the herb into pieces and boil with water for half an hour. Drink this as a tea.

Functions: Clears heat, eliminates vexation, and disinhibits the urine

Indications: This tea is suitable for the treatment of mouth and tongue sores, vexation of the heart, inhibited and painful urination, and dark-colored, *i.e.*, reddish, urine.

Radish Juice Mouth Rinse Tea (*Luo Bo Zhi Su Kou Cha*)

Radish, *i.e.*, Radix Raphani Sativi (*Luo Bo*)   1 radish

Method of administration: Wash the radish well, chop it into pieces, and then pound well to extract the juice. Rinse mouth with the radish juice a few times per day.

Functions: Dissipates static blood, disperses accumulation and stagnation, and eliminates heat and toxins

Indications: This tea is suitable for the treatment of mouth and tongue sores and oral putrescence.

Gum Inflammation Tea

Periodontitis or gum inflammation is a common disease affecting the soft tissues surrounding the teeth. The signs are gingival or gum bleeding, redness, swelling, inflammation, pain or sensitivity, or even a small amount of suppuration overflowing around the teeth. Inflammation of the gums in TCM is usually due to either replete heat in the liver and stomach or vacuity heat due to yin vacuity below.

Toothache Tea (*Ya Tong Cha*)

Rhubarb root, *i.e.*, Radix Et Rhizoma Rhei (*Da Huang*)   15 grams

Uncooked Gypsum (*Sheng Shi Gao*)   30 grams

Method of administration: Place these two herbs in a cup and steep in boiling water. They may be resoaked 2-3 times. Use 1 packet per day, once in the morning and again in the evening.

Functions: Clears heat and drains fire

Indications: This tea is suitable for the treatment of gastritis, toothache, and tooth bed putrefaction and bleeding due to replete heat in the *yang ming*.

Contraindications: This tea is contraindicated in individuals with weak constitutions and during pregnancy. While using these herbs, smoking, drinking alcohol, and eating greasy and fried foods are forbidden.

Tooth Decay Teas

Tooth decay or dental caries is a very common disease that can affect anyone. However, it is most common among children and the elderly. It is the major cause of toothache and tooth damage.

Fortify the Teeth Tea (*Jian Chi Cha*)

Tea leaves, *i.e.*, Folium Camelliae Theae (*Cha Ye*)   1-3 grams

Method of administration: Place the Tea leaves in a cup and steep in boiling water. Drink this while it is warm. Drink 1-2 cups per day. After drinking, rinse the mouth with Tea water also.

Functions: Removes the rotten and eliminates dental decay, cleans the teeth and prevents tooth decay

Indications: This tea is suitable for preventing and treating tooth decay and disease in the oral cavity.

218

Daphne, Asarum, Szechuan Pepper & Mugwort Tea (*Yuan Xin Jiao Ai Cha*)

Flos Daphnis Genkwae (*Yuan Hua*)   Equal amounts of each herb
Herba Asari Cum Radice (*Xi Xin*)
Szechuan pepper, *i.e.*, Fructus Zanthoxyli Bungeani (*Chuan Jiao*)
Mugwort, *i.e.*, Folium Artemisiae Argyii (*Ai Ye*)
Blighted wheat , *i.e.*, Fructus Levis Tritici Aestivi (*Fu Xiao Mai*)
Fine Tea, *i.e.*, Folium Camelliae Theae (*Xi Cha*)

Method of administration: Boil equal amounts of the above herbs with 250-500ml of water until 150-300ml of liquid is left. Use the warm liquid to rinse the mouth 3-4 times per day. When drooling occurs after rinsing the mouth with this tea, then the condition is cured. Do not drink or swallow the liquid.

Functions: Dispels wind, kills worms, and stops pain

Indications: This tea is suitable for the treatment of decayed teeth and toothache caused by vacuity fire.

Contraindications: This formula is a mouth rinse only and is not to be ingested.

Laryngitis Teas

There are two types of laryngitis—acute and chronic. The acute type refers to a redness and swelling of an area of the mucous membranes of the throat. This is referred to as "throat bi" in TCM. The chronic type is usually develops gradually from the acute type. Individuals with chronic rhinitis and nasal sinusitis also tend to have chronic laryngitis due to nasal congestion and from breathing through the mouth or due to purulent secretion irritating the naso-laryngeal area.

Sterculia Tea (*Pang Da Hai Cha*)

Semen Sterculiae Scaphageriae (*Pang Da Hai*)   3 pieces
Honey (*Feng Mi*)   15 grams

Method of administration: Place the herb into a teacup, add the honey, and pour in boiling water. Cover the cup for 3-4 minutes, open, and stir well with a spoon. Drink this freely as a tea.

Functions: Clears heat and moistens the lungs, disinhibits the throat and resolves toxins

Indications: This tea is suitable for the treatment of sore throat, dry cough without phlegm, a hoarse voice, bone-steaming with internal heat, hemoptysis and spontaneous external bleeding, red eye, toothache, hemorrhoids, and fistula.

Clear the Throat Tea (*Qing Yan Cha*)

Honeysuckle flower, *i.e.*, Flos Lonicerae Japonicae (*Jin Yin Hua*)   9 grams
Radix Scrophulariae Ningpoensis (*Xuan Shen*)   9 grams
Chinese olives, *i.e.*, Fructus Canarii (*Qing Guo*)   9 grams

Method of administration: Boil these three ingredients with water and strain off the liquids. Drink the resulting liquid repeatedly as a tea, 1 packet per day.

Functions: Clears heat and nourishes yin, resolves toxins and disinhibits the throat

Indications: This tea is suitable for the treatment of chronic laryngitis.

Laryngitis Tea (*Yan Yan Cha*)

Wild chrysanthemum flower, *i.e.*, Flos Chrysanthemum Indici
   (*Ye Ju Hua*)   12 grams

Tuber Ophiopogonis Japonici (*Mai Men Dong*)   12 grams
Honeysuckle flower, *i.e.*, Flos Lonicerae Japonicae (*Jin Yin Hua*) 12 grams

Method of administration: Place the above herbs into a teapot and steep in boiling water. Drink this as a tea, using 1 packet per day. It can be resoaked 3-4 times.

Functions: Clears heat and engenders fluids

Indications: This tea is suitable for the treatment of acute and chronic laryngitis.

Soothe the Throat Tea (*Shu Yan Cha*)

Semen Sterculiae Scaphigeriae (*Pang Da Hai*)   9 grams
Radix Platycodi Grandiflori (*Jie Geng*)   5 grams
Uncooked licorice root, *i.e.*, Radix Glycyrrhizae Uralensis
   (*Sheng Gan Cao*)   5 grams

Method of administration: Place the above herbs in a container. Soak with boiled water and cover for 10 minutes. Use 1 packet per day. Drink this as a tea.

Functions: Clears the lungs and disinhibits the throat

Indications: This tea is suitable for the treatment of chronic laryngitis and laryngeal discomfort caused by various factors.

Clear the Throat & Normalize the Qi Tea (*Qing Yan Shun Qi Cha*)

Field mint or peppermint, *i.e.*, Herba Menthae Haplocalycis (*Bo He*) 5 grams
Green Tea, *i.e.*, Folium Camelliae Theae (*Lu Cha*)   5 grams
Borneol (*Bing Pian*)   0.2 grams

Method of administration: Place these three ingredients in a cup. Soak with boiling water for 3 minutes and then drink.

Functions: Clears heat and engenders liquid, disperses food and descends the qi

Indications: This tea is suitable for the treatment of acute and chronic laryngopharyngitis, abdominal distention and fullness, and unexpelled flatulence.

Arhat Fruit Tea (*Luo Han Guo Cha*)

Arhat fruit, *i.e.*, Fructus Momordicae Grosvenori (*Luo Han Guo*) 10-15 grams
Green Tea, *i.e.*, Folium Camelliae Theae (*Lu Cha*)   1 gram

Method of administration: Chop the arhat fruit into pieces and then soak with the green Tea in boiling water. Cover for 5 minutes and then drink.

Functions: Clears heat and transforms phlegm, moistens the throat and stops thirst

Indications: This tea is suitable for the treatment of phlegm fire and sore throat.

Lophatherum & Ophiopogon Tea (*Zhu Ye Mai Dong Cha*)

Fresh Herba Lophatheri Gracilis (*Xian Dan Zhu Ye*)   10-15 sheets
Tuber Ophiopogonis Japonici (*Mai Men Dong*)   6 grams
Green Tea, *i.e.*, Folium Camelliae Theae (*Lu Cha*)   1 gram

Method of administration: Cut the two herbs into slices and place them with the Tea into a cup. Soak with boiled water, cover for 10 minutes, and drink.

Functions: Clears heat and nourishes yin, engenders fluids and stops thirst

Indications: This tea is suitable for the treatment of lung heat pattern chronic laryngopharyngitis.

Olive Tea (*Gan Lan Cha*)

Chinese olives, *i.e.*, Fructus Canarii (*Gan Lan*)	5-6 pieces
Crystal sugar (*Bing Tang*)	Amount to taste

Method of administration: Place the olives in a cup, add the crystal sugar, and pour in boiling water. Drink this repeatedly as a tea.

Functions: Clears the lungs and disinhibits the throat, engenders fluids and resolves toxins

Indicatons: This tea is suitable for the treatment of chronic laryngo-pharyngitis.

Western Olive Tea (*Xi Qing Guo Cha*)

Western olives (*Xi Qing Guo*)	6 pieces

Method of administration: Rinse the olives and then pound into pieces. Soak with boiled water. Drink the resulting liquid repeatedly as a tea.

Functions: Clears heat and engenders fluids, disinhibits the throat and resolves toxins, opens the voice and astringes the intestines

Indications: This tea is suitable for the treatment of chronic laryngitis and pharyngitis.

Olive, Lophatherum & Umeboshi Tea (*Lan Zhu Mei Cha*)

Salty olives, *i.e.*, salty Fructus Canarii (*Xian Gan Lan*)	5 pieces

223

Herba Lophatheri Gracilis (*Dan Zhu Ye*)   5 grams
Green Tea, *i.e.*, Folium Camelliae Theae (*Lu Cha*)   5 grams
Umeboshi, *i.e.*, Fructus Pruni Mume (*Wu Mei*)   2 pieces
White sugar (*Bai Tang*)   10 grams

Method of administration: Boil these five ingredients with water and drink the resulting liquid warm. Use 2 packets per day. One packet makes 1 cup of tea.

Functions: Clears the lungs and moistens the throat

Indications: This tea is suitable for the treatment of chronic cough, loss of voice due to exhaustion, and acute and chronic laryngopharyngitis.

Sterculia & Uncooked Rehmannia Tea (*Da Hai Sheng Di Cha*)

Semen Sterculiae Scaphageriae (*Pang Da Hai*)   12 grams
Uncooked Radix Rehmanniae (*Sheng Di*)   12 grams
Crystal sugar (*Bing Tang*)   30 grams

Method of administration: Place the two herbs and the sugar into a container and soak with boiled water. Drink the resulting liquid as a tea.

Functions: Opens and diffuses the lungs, enriches yin and cools the blood

Indications: This tea is suitable for the treatment of hoarse voice due to yin vacuity.

Terminalia & Ophiopogon Tea (*He Zi Mai Dong Cha*)

Fructus Terminaliae Chebulae (*He Zi*)   3 grams
Tuber Ophiopogonis Japonici (*Mai Men Dong*)   6 grams
Semen Oroxyli Indici (*Mu Hu Die*)   2 grams
Semen Sterculiae Scaphageriae (*Pang Da Hai*)   2 pieces

Method of administration: Soak the above four herbs together with boiled water and then drink.

Functions: Nourishes yin and clears the lungs, engenders fluids and opens the voice

Indications: This tea is suitable for the treatment of voice loss due to lung heat and yin vacuity.

Sterculia, Honey & Olive Tea (*Hai Mi Gan Lan Cha*)

Green Tea, *i.e.*, Folium Camelliae Theae (*Lu Cha*)	6 grams
Olive, *i.e.*, Fructus Canarii (*Gan Lan*)	6 grams
Semen Sterculiae Scaphigeriae (*Pang Da Hai*)	3 pieces
Honey (*Feng Mi*)	1 spoonful

Method of administration: First boil the olives with a suitable amount of clear water. Then use the boiled liquid to soak the green Tea and sterculia seeds. Cover with a lid for a short time and then add in the honey and stir well. Drink slowly.

Functions: Clears fire and disperses inflammation

Indications: This tea is suitable for the treatment of chronic laryngitis with a hoarse voice and a dry, sore throat.

Plum Pit Qi Teas

Plum pit qi is a TCM disease category similar to the symptoms of chronic laryngitis. It also covers neurotic esophageal stenosis or globus hystericus. Clinically, its main symptom is a discomfort in the throat area as if there were a piece of meat or a plum pit stuck in the back of the throat which can neither be spit up or swallowed down. Other accompanying symptoms include glomus and oppression in the chest and lateral costal regions, qi depression and inhibition, hiccough, and nausea. This condition is more common among women than among men and, therefore, some TCM books list this as a miscellaneous gynecological disease. If no obvious organic pathology can be found, the following tea formulas may be used based on the individual's pattern discrimination and signs and symptoms. However, since this condition is closely tied to emotional factors, the person should be counseled on stress reduction and relaxation.

Magnolia & Citron Tea (*Po Fo Cha*)

Flos Magnoliae Officinalis (*Hou Po Hua*)	6 grams
Flos Citri Sacrodactylis (*Fo Shou Hua*)	12 grams

Note: This medicinal is *not* the same as Flos Magnoliae Liliflorae (*Xin Yi Hua*).

Method of administration: Steep these two ingredients in boiling water for 10 minutes. Drink the tea slowly and take for 2-3 weeks con- tinuously.

Functions: Courses the liver and opens depression, downbears counterflow and rectifies the qi

Indications: This tea is suitable for the treatment of liver qi depression and binding due to inhibited emotion with phlegm and qi mutual obstruction which causes plum pit qi symptoms without any detectable redness or swelling in the throat.

Two Flowers Codonopsis & Barley Tea (*Er Hua Shen Mai Cha*)

Flos Magnoliae Officinalis (*Hou Po Hua*)	3 grams
Flos Citri Sacrodactylis (*Fo Shou Hua*)	3 grams
Black Tea, *i.e.*, prepared Folium Camelliae Theae (*Hong Cha*)	3 grams
Tangerine veins, *i.e.,* Fasciculus Vascularis Citri Reticulatae (*Ju Luo*)	2 grams

Radix Codonopsitis Pilosulae (*Dang Shen*)   6 grams
Stir-fried malted barley, *i.e.*, stir-fried Fructus Germinatus
   Hordei Vulgaris (*Chao Mai Ya*)   6 grams

Method of administration: Grind all the above ingredients into a coarse powder. Steep in boiling water and cover for 10 minutes. Use 1 packet per day. Drink the resulting liquid warm at any time.

Functions: Courses the liver and rectifies the qi, fortifies the spleen and disperses food, transforms phlegm and scatters nodulation

Indications: This tea is suitable for the treatment of unsmooth and depressed qi, phlegm and food accumulation, and plum pit qi complicated by spleen vacuity and food stagnation. In this case, there is a thick, slimy tongue coating and a slippery, wiry pulse. Other symptoms may include nausea, chest oppression, no thought for food, and possibly bad breath and belching.

Two Flowers Platycodon & Cornus Tea (*Er Hua Jie Zhu Cha*)

Flos Et Fructus Rosae Chinensis (*Yue Ji Hua*)   3 grams
Rose flower, *i.e.*, Flos Rosae Rugosae (*Mei Gui Hua*)   3 grams
Green Tea, *i.e.*, Folium Camelliae Theae (*Lu Cha*)   3 grams
Radix Platycodi Grandiflori (*Jie Geng*)   6 grams
Fructus Corni Officinalis (*Shan Zhu Yu*)   6 grams

Method of administration: Grind the above five ingredients into a coarse powder and steep in boiling water for 10 minutes. Use 1 packet per day. Drink this freely at any time. The medicinals may be resoaked several times.

Functions: Courses the liver and quickens the blood, nourishes yin and disinhibits the throat

Indications: This tea is suitable for the treatment of qi depression and blood stasis with depression and obstruction in the throat giving rise to the symptoms of plum pit qi.

Tangerine & Magnoliae Tea (*Ju Po Cha*)

Tangerine veins, *i.e.*, Fasciculus Vascularis Citri Reticulatae (*Ju Luo*) 3 grams
Cortex Magnoliae Officinalis (*Hou Po*)   3 grams
Black Tea, *i.e.*, prepared Folium Camelliae Theae (*Hong Cha*)   3 grams
Radix Codonopsitis Pilosulae (*Dang Shen*)   6 grams

Method of administration: Grind these four ingredients into a coarse powder. Place the powder in a container and steep in boiling water for 10 minutes. Use 1 packet per day, drink it at any time.

Functions: Courses the liver and rectifies the qi, resolves depression and transforms phlegm and dampness

Indications: This tea is suitable for the treatment of plum pit qi due to stagnant qi and phlegm dampness.

Dizziness Prevention Teas

In TCM, eye dizziness refers to vertigo, while head dizziness refers to a feeling of light-headedness such as in orthostatic hypotension or dizziness when standing up. Both may occur simultaneously. Therefore, they may be collectively called dizziness in the Chinese medical literature. In TCM, the causes of dizziness are yang vacuity with internal coldness, yang vacuity with water counterflow, ascendant liver yang, liver wind stirring internally, phlegm heat disturbing upward, or dual vacuity of qi and blood. In Western medicine, dizziness may be a symptom of Meniere's disease, hypertension, vestibular neuritis, or cerebellum disequilibrium.

Mulberry Leaf Tea (*Sang Ye Cha*)

Mulberry leaf, *i.e.*, Folium Mori Albi (*Sang Ye*)   10 grams
Chrysanthemum flower, *i.e.*, Flos Chrsanthemi Morifolii (*Ju Hua*) 10 grams
Fructus Lycii Chinensis (*Gou Qi Zi*)   10 grams

Semen Cassiae Torae (*Jue Ming Zi*)   6 grams

Method of administration: Boil the above ingredients and use the liquid. Drink this frequently as a tea.

Functions: Clears heat and dissipates wind, calms the liver and stabilizes dizziness

Indications: This tea is suitable for the treatment of head and eye dizziness due to stirring internally of liver wind.

Gastrodia Tea (*Tian Ma Cha*)

Rhizoma Gastrodiae Elatae (*Tian Ma*)   3-5 grams
Green Tea, *i.e.*, Folium Camelliae Theae (*Lu Cha*)   1 gram

Method of administration: Cut the gastrodia into thin slices and place in a cup with green Tea. Soak these in boiled water for 5 minutes and then drink. Use 1 packet per day.

Functions: Calms the liver and extinguishes fire, subdues yang and stabilizes fright

Indications: This tea is suitable for the treatment of dizziness and vertigo, tinnitus, a bitter taste in the mouth, fright and fear, numbness of the four limbs, paralysis of the limbs, and convulsive spasms of the limbs due to liver yang hyperactivity or depressive heat giving rise to internal stirring of wind. Taken over a long period of time, this formula is a good preventative for those at risk for stroke due to liver repletion.

Milk & Chrysanthemum Tea (*Nai Ju Cha*)

Cow's milk (*Niu Nai*)   1 cup
Chrysanthemum flower, *i.e.*, Flos Chrysanthemi Morifolii (*Ju Hua*)   20 flowers

229

White sugar (*Bai Tang*)   Amount to taste

Method of administration: Boil the milk and sugar together, add the chrysanthemum flowers, and bring to a second boil. Place the entire contents into a bowl and cover for a short time. Discard the dregs and drink the liquid. This can be taken hot or cool and may be stored in the refrigerator for later use as a cold drink.

Functions: Clears and disinhibits the head and eyes

Indications: This tea is suitable for the treatment of individuals who do mental work and use their eyes a lot, thus exhibiting a liver yin and blood vacuity with liver yang hyperactivity .

Sweet Chrysanthemum Tea (*Tian Ju Cha*)

Chrysanthemum flower, *i.e.*, Flos Chrysanthemi Morifolii (*Ju Hua*)   50 grams
Honey (*Feng Mi*)   250 grams

Method of administration: Place the chrysanthemum flowers into a pot, add 200ml of water, and boil for 25 minutes. When cool, discard the dregs, and use the liquid. Add honey to the liquid, stir well, and drink.

Functions: Nourishes the liver and moistens the lungs, brightens the eyes and arouses the brain

Indications: This tea is suitable for the treatment of headache, dizziness, swollen and sore throat, and constipation. Taken often, this formula promotes a cheerful spirit and restores youth.

Headache Teas

Headache is a common encountered condition in clinical practice and can be caused by a number of reasons. TCM divides headache into two categories: external contraction and internal damage. For external wind cold headache, the

230

symptoms are headache with aversion to cold and nasal congestion with a runny nose. For external wind heat headache, the symptoms are headache with aversion to wind, oral thirst, and a sore throat. For wind damp headache, the symptoms are headache with heaviness and aversion to the wind, a tight chest, and fatigue. For internal damage kidney vacuity headache, the symptoms are headache with dizziness, low back and knee soreness and weakness, or seminal emission. In liver effulgent headache, the headache occurs easily when there is anxiety, tiredness, or anger. Liver effulgent headaches are further divided into liver fire, liver yang, and liver wind headaches. For phlegm inversion headache, the symptoms are headache with dizziness, propping fullness in the chest and diaphragm, vomiting, and phlegm drool. For qi and blood vacuity, the symptoms are headache with vertigo, a lusterless facial complexion or pale lips and nails, and little taste for food or drink. The following tea formulas should, therefore, be used according to the individual's TCM pattern discrimination.

Ligusticum Tea (*Chuan Xiong Cha*)

Radix Ligustici Wallichii (*Chuan Xiong*)	3 grams
Radix Angelicae Dahuricae (*Bai Zhi*)	3 grams
Tea leaves, *i.e.*, Folium Camelliae Theae (*Cha Ye*)	6 grams

Method of administration: Grind the above ingredients into a fine powder. Place in a container and soak in boiled water. Take 1 packet per day.

Functions: Dispels wind and stops pain

Indications: This tea is suitable for the treatment of all conditions with wind attacking upward giving rise to symptoms such as dizziness, heavy head and eyes, unilateral or bilateral headache, nasal congestion, and bodily heaviness.

Ligusticum Wind Heat Headache Tea
(*Feng Re Tou Tong Chuan Xiong Cha*)

Radix Ligustici Wallichii (*Chuan Xiong*)	3 grams

Tea leaves, *i.e.*, Folium Camelliae Theae (*Cha Ye*)   6 grams

Method of administration: Boil these two herbs with 1 small bowl of water. Discard the dregs and use the liquid. Drink warm before meals, 2 packets per day.

Functions: Dispels wind and dissipates heat, rectifies the qi and stops pain

Indications: This tea is suitable for the treatment of wind heat headache.

Cassia Seed Tea (*Jue Ming Zi Cha*)

Semen Cassiae Torae (*Jue Ming Zi*)   100 grams

Method of administration: Stir-fry the herb and then grind into a powder. Mix this powder with Tea water and apply the powder to the acupuncture points on the temples, *i.e.*, *Tai Yang* (M-HN-3), changing this when it dries. Repeat many times.

Functions: Calms the liver and subdues yang

Indications: This tea is suitable for the treatment of liver yang headache. The symptoms of this type of headache are a pulling pain on the top of the head, dizziness, vexation and agitation, irascibility, and troubled sleep.

General Tea (*Jiang Jun Cha*)

Rhubarb root, *i.e.*, Radix Et Rhizoma Rhei (*Da Huang*)   A suitable amount
Tea leaves, *i.e.*, Folium Camelliae Theae (*Cha Ye*)   A suitable amount
Yellow rice or millet wine (*Huang Jiu*)   A suitable amount

Method of administration: Stir-fry the rhubarb with wine 3 times and then grind into a fine powder. When dry, place this powder in a container and seal. Each time, use 3-5 grams of this powder with 3 grams of Tea leaves by soaking both in boiling water. Drink warm, 1-2 times per day.

Functions: Clears heat and calms inversion, drains fire and stops pain

Indications: This tea is suitable for the treatment of heat inversion headache.

Contraindications: Stop taking this tea as soon as the pain stops so as to avoid injuring the righteous qi by long-term use of this formula. Rhubarb is contraindicated for use during pregnancy.

Silkworm & Scallion Tea (*Jiang Can Cong Bai Cha*)

Bombyx Batryticatus (*Jiang Can*)	A suitable amount
Scallion, *i.e.*, Bulbus Allii Fistulosi (*Cong Bai*)	6 grams
Green Tea, *i.e.,* Folium Camelliae Theae (*Lu Cha*)	3 grams

Method of administration: Dry bake the silkworm over a slow fire and then grind into a fine powder for later use. Each time use 3 grams of the above powder, boiling it, the green Tea, and the scallion with water. This may be taken 1-2 times per day.

Note: Batryticated silkworm purchased from Chinese herbal suppliers is already dried and ready for powdering.

Functions: Dispels wind and stops pain

Indications: This tea is suitable for unilateral or bilateral headache. It is also effective for chronic and headaches of year's duration.

Angelica Tea (*Bai Zhi Cha*)

Radix Angelicae Dahuricae (*Bai Zhi*)	10 grams
White sugar (*Bai Tang*)	Amount to taste

Method of administration: Boil the angelica with water, then add the sugar, and let it melt. Discard the dregs and drink.

Functions: Dispels wind and dampness and stops pain

Indications: This tea is suitable for wind damp headache. The symptoms of this type of headache are a headache that feels like a bandage wrapped around the head, tired and heavy limbs, a tight chest, scanty appetite, inhibited urination, or loose stools and diarrhea. There is a slimy, white tongue coating and a soggy pulse. The headache is worse especially in cloudy and damp weather.

Selfheal & Lotus Leaf Tea (*Xia Ku Cao He Ye Cha*)

Selfheal spike, *i.e.*, Spica Prunellae Vulgaris (*Xia Ku Cao*)	10 grams
Lotus leaf, *i.e.*, Folium Nelumbinis Nuciferae (*He Ye*)	12 grams

Note: If using fresh lotus leaf, use one half of a sheet.

Method of administration: Boil these two herbs with water. Discard the dregs and use the liquid.

Functions: Enriches the kidneys and calms the liver

Indications: This tea is suitable for liver/kidney yin vacuity and wind fire hyperactivity above. The symptoms of this type of headache are frequent headache and vertigo at no particular time, dizziness, tinnitus, possible sudden deviation of the eyes and mouth, stiffness of the tongue impeding speech, heavy, stagnant hands and feet, hemiplegia, a red tongue with a yellow coating, and a wiry, slippery, rapid pulse.

13
Cancers

The teas in this chapter are meant for adjunctive or supportive use only. They are not meant as comprehensive treatments for various types of cancers. The authors and publishers of this book strongly advise all persons with a confirmed or suspected diagnosis of cancer to seek treatment from well-trained and experienced professional medical practitioners. When used as part of a comprehensive medical treatment plan, these Chinese medicinal teas can be a useful addition. For more informaton on the Chinese medical treatment of cancer, readers should see Zhang Dai-zhao's *The Treatment of Cancer by Integrated Chinese-Western Medicine* published by Blue Poppy Press.

Nasopharyngeal Carcinoma Teas

The main symptoms for nasopharyngeal carcinoma are nasal obstruction, nasal bleeding, headache, tinnitus, ambiopia or double vision, and swollen lumps appearing in the nasopharyngeal area and the area under the ear. This is similar to "loss of luxuriance" condition in TCM and occurs commonly in southern China. Currently, Western medical treatments for this disease are radiation and chemotherapy. Based on experience in China combining traditional Chinese and modern Western medicines, the result of radiation and chemotherapy can be increased by combining those treatments with TCM herbal tea formulas.

Umeboshi Anticancer Tea (*Wu Mei Kang Ai Cha*)

Umeboshi, *i.e.*, Fructus Pruni Mume (*Wu Mei*)	25 grams
Green Tea, *i.e.*, Folium Cameliae Theae (*Lu Cha*)	2 grams
Licorice root, *i.e.*, Radix Glycyrrhizae Uralensis (*Gan Cao*)	5 grams

Method of administration: Boil the umeboshi and licorice in 800ml of water for 10 minutes. Then add the green Tea and boil for another minute. Drink the liquid. Use 1 packet per day taken in 3 divided doses.

Functions: Disperses inflammation and dispels phlegm, resolves toxins and combats cancer

Indications: This tea is suitable for the treatment of nasopharyngeal carcinoma and rectal carcinoma. Taken often, this tea can engender fluids and moisten the lungs, resolve toxins and combat cancer. It has fairly good results for restraining the development and metastasis of carcinoma cells.

Lithospermum Decocted Tea (*Zi Cao Jian Cha*)

Radix Lithopsermi Seu Arnebiae (*Zi Cao Gen*)   30 grams

Method of administration: Boil this herb with water. Drink the resulting liquid as a tea. Use 1 packet per day.

Functions: Clears heat and resolves toxins, cools the blood and stops bleeding

Indications: This tea is suitable for the treatment of nasopharyngeal carcinoma.

Pulmonary Carcinoma Teas

Pulmonary carcinoma is a common respiratory tract cancer. In TCM, pulmonary carcinoma falls under the traditional disease categories of "cough," "phlegm rheum," "inverted cup syndrome," and "hacking blood." Its clinical symptoms are a paroxysmal, irritating, dry cough with scanty, clear, watery phlegm streaked with blood or hacking up of blood, chest pain, chest opression, shortness of breath, fever, and a hoarse voice. Pulmonary cancer is divided into primary and metastatic types due to its different sites of origin. Presently in China, the dominant treatment method for the primary type of pulmonary carcinoma is surgery. A comprehensive treatment combining Western and Chinese medicine is typcially used for the treatment of metastatic or advanced stage lung cancer. This treatment includes radiation, chemotherapy, Chinese herbs, special diet, and medicinal teas.

Honeysuckle Anticancer Tea (*Yin Hua Kang Ai Cha*)

Honeysuckle flower, *i.e.*, Flos Lonicerae Japonicae (*Yin Hua*)   10-25 grams
Green Tea, *i.e.*, Folium Camelliae Theae (*Lu Cha*)   2 grams
Licorice root, *i.e.*, Radix Glycyrrhizae Uralensis (*Gan Cao*)   5 grams

Method of administration: Boil the honeysuckle flower and licorice in 500ml of water for 10 minutes. Add the green Tea and then boil for another half minute. Take 1 packet per day, drink it warm in 2 divided doses.

Functions: Clears heat, resolves toxins, and combats cancer

Indications: This tea is suitable for the treatment of pulmonary carcinoma and carcinoma of the stomach.

Trichosanthes Anticancer Tea (*Gua Lou Kang Ai Cha*)

Fructus Trichosanthis Kirlowii (*Gua Lou*)   5 grams
Green Tea, *i.e.*, Folium Camelliae Theae (*Lu Cha*)   2 grams
Licorice root, *i.e.*, Radix Glycyrrhizae Uralensis (*Gan Cao*)   3 grams

Method of administration: Boil the trichosanthes fruit and licorice in 600ml of water 5-10 minutes. Add the green Tea and boil for another 3 minutes. Drink 1 packet per day, once in the morning and again in the afternoon. When necessary, 2 packets can be taken in 1 day.

Functions: Combats cancer and moistens the lungs, dispels phlegm and loosens the chest, scatters nodulation

Indications: This tea is suitable for the treatment of pulmonary carcinoma with cough, chest oppression, and copious, hard to expectorate phlegm.

Houttuynia Tea (*Ji Cai Cha*)

Herba Houttuyniae Cordatae Cum Radice (*Yu Xing Cao*)	30 grams
Honeysuckle flower, *i.e.*, Flos Lonicerae Japonicae (*Jin Yin Hua*)	9 grams
Radix Scutellariae Baicalensis (*Huang Qin*)	9 grams
Green Tea, *i.e.*, Folium Camelliae Theae (*Lu Cha*)	3 grams
Honey (*Feng Mi*)	1 spoonful

Method of administration: Boil the first three ingredients with a suitable amount of water for 10 minutes. Add the green Tea and boil for another 3 minutes. Strain off the liquid and add honey. An alternate method is to dry the first four ingredients over a gentle heat and then grind them into powder. Steep in boiling water for 10 minutes and then add honey. Use 1 packet per day, taken at any time.

Functions: Combats cancer, clears heat and resolves toxins, moistens the lungs and transforms phlegm

Indications: This tea is suitable for the treatment of lung cancer with cough, copious phlegm streaked with blood, and a low-grade fever. It is especially for middle and advanced stage patients who cannot have surgery.

Dandelion & Green Tea (*Gong Ying Lu Cha*)

Green Tea, *i.e.*, Folium Camelliae Theae (*Lu Cha*)	2 grams
Dandelion, *i.e.*, Herba Taraxaci Mongolici Cum Radice (*Pu Gong Ying*)	15-25 grams
Licorice root, *i.e.*, Radix Glycyrrhizae Uralensis (*Gan Cao*)	3 grams
Honey (*Feng Mi*)	15 grams

Method of administration: Boil the dandelion and licorice in 500ml of water for 10 minutes. Add the green Tea and honey, bring to a boil again, and then take from heat. Drink the resulting liquid warm. Use 1 packet per day taken in 3 doses.

Functions: Clears heat and resolves toxins, disperses swelling and scatters nodulation, combats cancer

Indications: This tea is suitable for the treatment of pulmonary carcinoma.

Polyporus Tea (*Zhu Ling Cha*)

Sclerotium Polypori Umbellati (*Zhu Ling*)	10-25 grams
Green Tea, *i.e.*, Folium Camelliae Theae (*Lu Cha*)	2 grams
Licorice root, *i.e.*, Radix Glycyrrhizae Uralensis (*Gan Cao*)	5 grams

Method of administration: Pound the polyporus into pieces. Boil it and the licorice in 800ml of water for 10 minutes. Add the green Tea and bring it back to a boil. Then remove from the heat. Drink the resulting liquid warm. Use 1 packet per day taken in 3 doses.

Functions: Disinhibits water and transforms phlegm and dampness, resolves toxins and combats cancer

Indications: This tea is suitable for the treatment of pulmonary cancer and cancer of the esophagus.

Ginkgo & Job's Tears Barley Tea (*Bai Guo Yi Ren Cha*)

Semen Ginkgonis Bilobae (*Bai Guo Ren*)	8-12 pieces
Job's Tears barley, *i.e.*, Semen Coicis Lachryma-jobi (*Yi Yi Ren*)	100 grams
Crystal sugar or white sugar (*Bing Tang* or *Bai Tang*)	Amount to taste

239

Method of administration: Cook the first two ingredients thoroughly with water. Add sugar to taste and drink this as a tea.

Functions: Calms dyspnea or panting and expels pus, disperses pain and clears heat

Indications: This tea is suitable for the treatment of pulmonary cancer with constant dyspnea, cough, spleen vacuity diarrhea, dribbling painful urination, and water swelling.

Almond Tea (*Xing Ren Cha*)

Almond (*Tian Xing Ren*)	6 grams
Green Tea, *i.e.*, Folium Camelliae Theae (*Lu Cha*)	1 gram

Method of administration: Rinse the almonds in cold boiled water. Break into pieces, add 1,000ml of water, and boil over a medium fire. Use this liquid in place of water to make the green Tea. Cover for 5 minutes and then drink. Take 200ml every 3-4 hours.

Functions: Clears heat and moistens the lungs, resolves toxins and dispels phlegm, combats cancer

Indications: This tea has some effect for preventing of carcinomas of the lungs, breast, and intestines.

Asparagus Tea (*Tian Dong Cha*)

Tuber Asparagi Cochinensis (*Tian Men Dong*)	8 grams
Green Tea, *i.e.*, Folium Camelliae Theae (*Lu Cha*)	1 gram

Method of administration: Cut the asparagus tuber into pieces. Place these pieces in a cup, add the green Tea, and pour in boiling water. Cover the cup for 5 minutes and drink the tea at any time.

Functions: Moistens dryness and stops thirst, clears heat and transforms phlegm, combats germs and cancer

Indications: This tea has some effect for preventing lung and breast cancers.

Esophageal Carcinoma Teas

The symptoms of the initial stage of cancer of the esophagus are a substernal burning sensation, pain or food friction, and stagnating, obstructing, and choking sensations when swallowing food. In the beginning, these sensations are obvious only when eating hard food. Later, they gradually become persistent and progressive with the expectoration of frothy mucus. As the difficulty in swallowing increases and other symptoms develop, the patient's condition deteriorates quickly. The symptoms of emaciation, dehydration, constipation, and fatigue also increase. This disease belongs to the category of "constricted diaphragm" in TCM.

Clear the Stomach Tea (*Qing Wei Cha*)

Rhizoma Phragmitis Communis (*Lu Gen*)	50 pieces
Peach seed, *i.e.*, Semen Pruni Persicae (*Tao Ren*)	25 grams

Method of administration: Rinse and slice the phragmites. Place these slices into a pot and add water. Bring to a boil for 30 minutes over a gentle fire. Strain and reserve the liquid. Next, grind the peach seeds and stir into this liquid to make a thick drink. Use 1 packet per day taken in 2 doses.

Functions: Clears the stomach and downbears fire, breaks blood and scatters nodulation

Indications: This tea is suitable for the treatment of depressed, bound qi and fire in the blood causing esophageal constriction and stomach reflux.

Contraindications: This formula is not suitable for stomach reflux caused by spleen and stomach vacuity cold.

Fresh Chinese Leek Juice Tea (*Xian Jiu Cai Zhi Cha*)

Fresh Chinese leek, *i.e.*, Herba Alli Tuberosi (*Jiu Cai*)   A suitable amount
Cow's milk (*Niu Nai*)   1/2 cup

Method of administration: Pound the leeks to extract the juice. For each dose, mix 1 spoonful of this juice with warmed milk. Drink this slowly. This may be taken a few times each day.

Functions: Disinhibits the throat and harmonizes the stomach

Indications: This tea is suitable for the treatment of cancer of the esophagus.

Five Juices Quiet the Middle Tea (*Wu Zhi An Zhong Yin Cha*)

Chinese leek juice, *i.e.*, Succus Alli Tuberosi (*Jiu Cai Zhi*)
Cow's milk (*Niu Nai*)
Uncooked ginger juice, *i.e.*, uncooked Succus Rhizomatis Zingiberis
   (*Sheng Jiang Zhi*)
Pear juice, *i.e.*, Succus Pyri Communis (*Li Zhi*)
Lotus root juice, *i.e.*, Succus Rhizomatis Nelumbinis Nuciferae (*Ou Zhi*)
A suitable amount of each ingredient

Method of administration: Mix these five ingredients well and then drink as a tea at any time.

Functions: Disinhibits the throat, harmonizes the stomach, and moistens dryness

Indications: This tea is suitable for the treatment of esophageal constriction, dull pain, glomus and oppression in the chest and diaphragm, obstruction in

242

swallowing, a dry mouth and throat, difficult and inhibited defecation, and a withered body.

Ophiopogon & Uncooked Rehmannia Tea (*Mai Men Dong Sheng Di Huang Cha*)

Tuber Ophiopogonis Japonici (*Mai Men Dong*)	10 grams
Uncooked Radix Rehmanniae (*Sheng Di*)	15 grams
Lotus root juice, *i.e.*, Succus Rhizomatis Nelumbinis Nuciferae (*Ou Zhi*)	32 grams

Method of administration: Boil these herbs and the juice together. Remove the dregs and use the liquid. Drink as a tea.

Functions: Enriches yin, moistens dryness, and engenders fluids

Indications: This tea is suitable for the treatment of chronic esophageal constriction, emaciation, dry skin, and a pale facial complexion.

Clematis & Honey Tea (*Wei Ling Mi Zhi Cha*)

Honey (*Feng Mi*)	50 grams
Radix Clematidis Chinensis (*Wei Ling Xian*)	50 grams

Method of administration: Boil the above two ingredients with water and use the resulting liquid. Take 1 packet per day, once in the morning and again in the evening.

Functions: Moistens dryness and engenders fluids, softens the hard and transforms cancerous swelling

Indications: This tea is suitable as a supplementary treatment of cancer of the esophagus.

Goat's Milk Tea (*Yang Ru Cha*)

Goat's milk (*Yang Ru*)	250 grams
Bamboo juice, *i.e.*, Succus Bambusae (*Zhu Li Shui*)	20 grams
Honey (*Feng Mi*)	20 grams
Chinese leek juice, *i.e.*, Succus Alli Tuberosi (*Jiu Cai Zhi*)	10 grams

Method of administration: Boil the goat's milk first. Then add the bamboo juice, honey, and Chinese leek juice. Stir them well and drink this repeatedly at any time.

Functions: Warms yang and boosts the qi, disinhibits the diaphragm and harmonizes the stomach

Indications: This tea is suitable for the treatment of yang qi insufficiency in the elderly and congealed and bound phlegm and blood causing esophageal constriction and stomach reflux.

Gastric Carcinoma Teas

Gastric carcinoma or cancer of the stomach is a common cancer of the digestive tract. It belongs to the categories of "stomach pain," "stomach reflux," and "hiccough" in TCM. Its Western medical treatment typically includes surgery, radiation, and chemotherapy. From the TCM point of view, one should also treat the whole person based on their individualized TCM pattern discrimination. The following adjunctive tea formulas for stomach cancer should be chosen on the basis of such a pattern discrimination.

Job's Tears Barley Anticancer Tea (*Yi Ren Kang Ai Cha*)

Job's Tears barley, *i.e.*, Coicis Lachryma-jobi (*Yi Yi Ren*)	60 grams
Red dates, *i.e.*, Fructus Zizyphi Jujubae (*Hong Zao*)	30 grams
Green Tea, *i.e.*, Folium Camelliae Theae (*Lu Cha*)	3 grams

244

Method of administration: Steep the green Tea in boiling water for 5 minutes and set aside. Add fresh water to the Job's Tears and the chopped red dates and cook them into a kind of paste. Then add the Tea water to this paste. Use 1 packet per day. Drink this warm in 3 doses. One may drink the juice and also eat the two herbal ingredients.

Functions: Fortifies the spleen and disinhibits dampness, resolves toxins and transforms turbidity, combats cancerous tumors

Indications: This tea is suitable for the treatment of cancer of the stomach, cancer of the bladder, and cancer of the intestines.

Atractylodes Anticancer Tea (*Bai Zhu Kang Ai Cha*)

Green Tea, *i.e.*, Folium Camelliae Theae (*Lu Cha*)	2 grams
Rhizoma Atractylodis Macrocephalae (*Bai Zhu*)	9-15 grams
Licorice root, *i.e.*, Radix Glycyrrhizae Uralensis (*Gan Cao*)	3 grams

Method of administration: Add the licorice and atractylodes together in 600ml of water and boil for 10 minutes. Add the green Tea and boil all the ingredients for another minute. Strain off the liquid. Use 1 packet per day. Drink the resulting liquid warm in 3 doses daily.

Functions: Fortifies the spleen and boosts the qi, dries dampness and harmonizes the middle, combats cancer

Indications: This tea is suitable for the treatment of cancer of the stomach and cancer of the esophagus.

Tangerine Peel & Red Date Tea (*Ju Pi Hong Zao Cha*)

Tangerine peel, *i.e.*, Percarpium Citri Reticulatae (*Ju Pi*)	1 piece
Red dates, *i.e.*, Fructus Zizyphi Jujubae (*Hong Zao*)	3 pieces

Method of administration: Remove the red date seeds. Then boil the two ingredients with water. Drink the resulting liquid repeatedly at any time.

Functions: Moves the qi and fortifies the spleen, downbears counterflow and stops vomiting

Indications: This tea is suitable for the treatment of cancer of the stomach and vacuity cold type vomiting.

Sugarcane & Ginger Beverage Tea (*Zhe Jiang Yin Cha*)

Sugarcane (*Gan Zhe*)
Uncooked ginger, *i.e.,* uncooked Rhizoma Zingiberis Officinalis
   (*Sheng Jiang*)   A suitable amount of each

Method of administration: Extract a 1/2 cup of juice from the sugarcane and 1 teaspoonful of juice from the ginger. Mix together and warm with hot water. Use 1 packet per day.

Functions: Harmonizes the middle and fortifies the stomach

Indications: This tea is suitable for the treatment of the initial stage of stomach cancer, constant dry vomiting, and vomiting at night of food eaten in the morning.

Garlic Tea (*Da Suan Cha*)

Green Tea, *i.e.,* Folium Camelliae Theae (*Lu Cha*)	1.5 grams
Garlic bulb, *i.e.,* Bulbus Alli Sativi (*Da Suan Tou*)	9-25 grams
Brown sugar (*Hong Tang*)	25 grams

Method of administration: Peel the skin off of the garlic and pound into a paste. Mix the garlic with the green Tea and brown sugar. Steep in 500ml of boiled water for 10 minutes and drink. Use 1 packet per day. The ingredients can be resteeped 2-3 times per day and taken at any time.

246

Functions: Disperses inflammation and kills germs, clears heat and resolves toxins, combats cancerous tumors

Indications: This tea is suitable for the treatment of cancer of the stomach, cancer of the esophagus, and cancer of the breast.

Licorice & Peony Tea (*Gan Cao Hang Shao Cha*)

Licorice root, *i.e.*, Radix Glycyrrhizae Uralensis (*Gan Cao*)   20 grams
White peony root, *i.e.*, Radix Albus Paeoniae Lactiflorae (*Bai Shao*)   30 grams

Method of administration: Boil the above two ingredients with water and drink as a tea repeatedly.

Functions: Clears heat and resolves toxins, relaxes cramping and stops pain

Indications: This tea is suitable for the treatment of cancer of the stomach with pain.

Primary Liver Carcinoma Teas

In TCM, primary carcinoma of the liver is categorized as "spleen accumulation," "liver accumulation," "concretions and accumulations," "drum distention," and "jaundice." In the initial stage, surgery is the usual treatment. In the middle stage, hepatic artery catheterization with drug perfusion, radiation therapy, and chemotherapy are often used. In the advanced stage, comprehensive treatment with a combination of Chinese and Western medicine is typically considered necessary in China.

Artemisia Capillaris & Oldenlandia Tea (*Yin Chen She She Cao Cha*)

Herba Artemesiae Capillaris (*Yin Chen Hao*)   30 grams
Herba Oldenlandiae Diffusae (*Bai Hua She She Cao*)   30 grams
Licorice root, i.e., Radix Glycyrrhizae Uralensis (*Gan Cao*)   6 grams

Green Tea, *i.e.*, Folium Camelliae Theae (*Lu Cha*)	3 grams

Method of administration: Boil the first three herbs in 1,000ml of water for 15 minutes. Use the resulting liquid to infuse the green Tea. Use 1 packet per day. One may drink this slowly at any time.

Functions: Clears heat and transforms dampness, resolves toxins and removes jaundice, combats cancerous tumors

Indications: This tea is suitable for the treatment of carcinoma of the liver, especially when accompanied by ascites, jaundice, and cirrhosis of the liver. This formula can also be used for both the prevention and improvement of liver carcinoma.

Artemisia Capillaris & Brown Sugar Tea (*Yin Chen Hong Tang Cha*)

Herba Artemesiae Capillaris (*Yin Chen Hao*)	15 grams
Brown sugar (*Hong Tang*)	60 grams

Method of administration: Boil these two ingredients with water and drink as a tea repeatedly. Use 1 packet per day.

Functions: Clears heat and disinhibits dampness, abates jaundice

Indications: This tea is suitable for the treatment of carcinoma of the liver with jaundice as the main symptom.

Two Whites Beverage Tea (*Er Bai Yin Cha*)

Herba Oldenlandiae Diffusae (*Bai Hua She She Cao*)	100 grams
Rhizoma Imperatae Cylindricae (*Bai Mao Gen*)	30 grams
White sugar (*Bai Tang*)	Amount to taste

Method of administration: Wash the two herbs well and place them in a pot. Add water and boil. Strain the liquid, add white sugar, and drink. Use 1 packet per day taken in 3 doses.

Functions: Clears heat and resolves toxins, cools the blood and engenders fluids

Indications: This tea has the effect of slowing down the symptoms of liver carcinoma.

Intestinal & Rectal Carcinoma Tea

Cancer of the intestines and rectum belongs to the category of "visceral toxins," "anus-locking hemorrhoids," "accumulations and gatherings," and "intestine egg" in TCM. Common symptoms are emaciation, a pale face, poor appetite, depression, fatigue, a downward sagging feeling in the abdomen, paroxysmal pain, drum distention, borborygmus, constipation, or alternating constipation and diarrhea. The stools are similar to goat feces or are like extruded, thin strips. The stool contains occult blood or mucus. Rectal cancer includes not only the above symptoms but also the symptoms of a sharp itching in the anus and tenesmus. In the advanced stage, fecal incontinence can occur due to the cancerous tumor affecting the sphincter muscle.

Coptis & Lotus Seed Tea (*Huang Lian Lian Zi Cha*)

Rhizoma Coptidis Chinensis (*Huang Lian*)	10 grams
Lotus seed, *i.e.*, Semen Nelumbinis Nuciferae (*Lian Zi*)	30 grams
Radix Codonopsitis Pilosulae (*Dang Shen*)	15 grams

Method of administration: Boil these three ingredients in water. Use 1 packet per day taken in 2 doses.

Functions: Clears heat and dries dampness, drains fire and resolves toxins

Indications: This tea is suitable for the treatment of cancer of the intestines accompanied by the symptoms of abdominal cramping and rectal heaviness.

Urinary Bladder Carcinoma Teas

Cancer of the urinary bladder is a common urological system tumor. It commonly affects men between the ages of 50-70. The main symptoms are bloody urination without pain and inhibited urination. Similar descriptions in the Chinese medical literature can be found under the disease categories of "bloody urine" and "bloody strangury." In its early and middle stages, surgery, radiation therapy, chemotherapy, and Chinese herbs should be taken. In the advanced stage, if surgery is unsuitable and radiation therapy can be delayed, then chemotherapy can be used according to the condition with Chinese medicinal herbs used as the dominant treatment methods.

Imperata & Job's Tears Barley Tea (*Mao Gen Mi Ren Cha*)

Rhizoma Imperatae Cylindricae (*Bai Mao Gen*)	30 grams
Job's Tears barley, *i.e.*, Semen Coicis Lachryma-jobi (*Yi Yi Ren*)	30 grams
Herba Oldenlandiae Diffusae (*Bai Hua She She Cao*)	15 grams
Green Tea, *i.e.*, Folium Camelliae Theae (*Lu Cha*)	3 grams

Method of administration: Boil the first three ingredients with 1,000ml of water for 15-20 minutes. They can be boiled twice. Discard the dregs and mix the liquid from the two boilings together with the green Tea. Use 1 packet per day. Drink this freely as a tea.

Functions: Clears heat and disinhibits dampness, cools the blood and stops bleeding, combats cancer

Indications: This tea is suitable for the treatment of urinary bladder carcinoma with blood in the urine. This formula is suitable for both the prevention and treatment of bladder cancer in the initial stage. It can also be used as an adjunctive method after surgery.

Pyrrosia Tea (*Shi Wei Cha*)

Folium Pyrrosiae (*Shi Wei*)	15 grams
Green Tea, *i.e.*, Folium Camelliae Theae (*Lu Cha*)	3 grams
Crystal sugar (*Bing Tang*)	25 grams

Method of administration: Place the pyrrosia leaves in a pot, add 500ml of water, and boil for 10 minutes. Add the green Tea and crystal sugar and then boil for 1 more minute. Strain the liquid and drink. Use 1 packet per day taken in 2 doses, 1 in the morning and 1 in the afternoon.

Functions: Clears heat and resolves toxins, disinhibits dampness and frees strangury, combats cancer

Indications: This tea is suitable for the treatment of cancer of the bladder. Taken often, this tea is effective for both preventing the occurrence of bladder cancer or improving the disease condition once it has occured.

Cervical Carcinoma Teas

Carcinoma of the uterine cervix is a relatively common female malignant tumor with most of the cases occurring between 40-60 years of age. Its main symptom is vaginal bleeding. In the early stage, bleeding after sexual intercourse is often seen. When the cancer reaches the middle and advanced states, symptoms of irregular vaginal bleeding, copious vaginal discharge like rice washing water with a fishy and foul smell, and low back and abdominal pain are often seen. Due to its various manifestations at different stages, this disease's description is scattered in the Chinese medical literature under the categories of "uterine bleeding," "vaginal discharge," and "concretions and conglomerations." Its Western medical treatment is usually cryosurgery or surgery combined with radiation and chemotherapy. Chinese herbal medicine can also be used for a comprehensive treatment of not only the disease symptoms but also the entire pattern of disharmony.

Ginkgo & Wax Gourd Seed Tea (*Bai Guo Dong Gua Zi Cha*)

Semen Ginkgonis Bilobae (*Bai Guo*)	10 pieces
Chinese wax gourd seed, *i.e.*, Semen Benincasae Hispidae (*Dong Gua Zi*)	30 grams
Lotus seed, *i.e.*, Semen Nelumbinis Nuciferae (*Lian Zi*)	15 grams
Black pepper, *i.e.*, Fructus Piperis Nigri (*Hu Jiao*)	1.5 grams

Method of administration: Boil the above herbs with water. Use 1 packet per day, drunk warm as a tea.

Functions: Fortifies the spleen, disinhibits dampness, and stops discharge

Indications: This tea is suitable for the treatment of carcinoma of the uterine cervix with constant vaginal discharge due to a combination of spleen vacuity and damp heat.

Black Cohosh & Green Tea (*Sheng Ma Lu Cha*)

Green Tea, *i.e.*, Folium Camelliae Theae (*Lu Cha*)	1.5 grams
Honey mix-fried black cohosh, *i.e.*, honey mix-fried Rhizoma Cimicifugae (*Mi Zhi Sheng Ma*)	5-15 grams
Mix-fried licorice root, *i.e.,* mix-fried Radix Glycyrrhizae Uralensis (*Zhi Gan Cao*)	10 grams

Method of administration: Boil these three ingredients in 400ml of water for 5-10 minutes. Use 1 packet per day taken in 3 doses after meals.

Functions: Clears heat and resolves toxins, combats cancerous tumors

Indications: This tea is suitable for the treatment of carcinoma of the uterine cervix. Taken often, this tea can help prevent uterine cervical inflammation, uterine cervical erosion, and carcinoma of the uterine cervix.

Breast Cancer Teas

Breast cancer is the most common malignant tumor among women. It is called "mammary rock" in TCM. Presently in China, its dominant treatment is surgery. Based on Chinese experience, better results can be achieved when surgery is combined with radiation, chemotherapy, Chinese herbal medicine, food therapy, and medicinal teas.

Asparagus & Fritillaria Tea (*Dong Bei Cha*)

Tuber Asparagi Cochinensis (*Tian Men Dong*)	30 grams
Earth-fried Bulbus Fritillariae (*Tu Chao Bei Mu*)	10 grams
Green Tea, *i.e.*, Folium Camelliae Theae (*Lu Cha*)	3 grams
Honey (*Feng Mi*)	1 teaspoon

Method of administration: Boil the first two herbs with water for 15 minutes. Use the liquid to brew the green Tea. Add in 1 teaspoon of honey. Drink 1 packet per day at any time.

Functions: Nourishes yin and moistens the lungs, clears heat and resolves toxins, disperses tumors and combats cancer

Indications: This tea is suitable for the treatment of breast cancer manifesting a pattern of yin vacuity and phlegm nodulation. Typically, breast lumps are seen as a type of phlegm nodulation in TCM. Radiation and chemotherapy also tend to damage and exhaust yin fluids by causing evil heat. Therefore, it is not uncommon to see women with breast cancer exhibiting this pattern of yin vacuity/vacuity heat with phlegm nodulation.

Asparagus & Brown Sugar Tea (*Tian Dong Hong Tang Cha*)

Tuber Asparagi Cochinensis (*Tian Men Dong*)	30 grams
Brown sugar (*Hong Tang*)	Amount to taste

Method of administration: Boil the asparagus with 2 bowls of clear water until only 1 bowl of liquid remains. Add the brown sugar and bring the mixture back to a boil. Drink this warm, 1 packet per day. An effect will typically be seen after 4 consecutive doses.

Functions: Nourishes yin and moistens the lungs

Indications: This tea is suitable for the treatment of hyperplasia of the lobule of the mammary gland and as a preventative for breast cancer in women exhibiting a pattern of yin vacuity. Yin vacuity signs and symptoms also commonly manifest during and after menopause, the time when women are most at risk for developing breast cancer.

Leukemia Teas

Cancer originating from the marrow and lymphatic system is called leukemia. Because of the disproportionate number of white blood cells in this disease, in Chinese it is called white blood disease. Descriptions similar to leukemia can be found under the headings "vacuity taxation," "acute taxation," "heat taxation," and "blood condition" in TCM. In Western medicine, leukemia is divided into acute lymphoblastic, acute nonlymphoblastic, chronic myelocytic, and chronic lymphocytic. The main symptoms of acute leukemia are bleeding, a pale complexion, and fever. The main symptoms of chronic leukemia are fatigue, lack of strength, poor appetite, weight loss, fever, night sweats, and abdominal fullness, while pallor and bleeding are unusual. As the disease progresses, there is enlargement of the spleen and lymphadenopathy.

Lophatherum & Imperata Beverage Tea (*Zhu Mao Yin Cha*)

Herba Lophatheri Gracilis (*Dan Zhu Ye*)	10 grams
Rhizoma Imperatae Cylindricae (*Bai Mao Gen*)	10 grams

Method of administration: Place these two herbs in a container, steep them in boiling water, and cover for 30 minutes. Use 1 packet per day. The same packet may be steeped and used repeatedly.

Functions: Clears heat and disinhibits water, cools the blood and stops bleeding

Indications: This tea is suitable for the treatment of leukemia with obvious blood in the urine.

Lotus Leaf & Node Decocted Tea (*He Ye Ou Jie Jian Cha*)

Fresh lotus leaf, *i.e.*, fresh Folium Nelumbinis Nuciferae
    (*Xian He Ye*)   One big sheet
Nodus Rhizomatis Nelumbinis Nuciferae (*Ou Jie*)   A couple nodes

Method of administration: Burn the lotus node until it is charred. Boil this with the lotus leaf in water. Strain and use the liquid. Use 1 packet per day. The same packet may be steeped repeatedly.

Functions: Clears heat, cools the blood, and stops bleeding

Indications: This tea is suitable for the treatment of leukemia with severe nosebleed.

Red Peony Tea (*Chi Shao Cha*)

Green Tea, *i.e.*, Folium Camelliae Theae (*Lu Cha*)   2 grams
Red peony root, *i.e.*, Radix Rubrus Paeoniae Lactiflorae
    (*Chi Shao*)   9-15 grams
Licorice root, *i.e.*, Radix Glycyrrhizae Uralensis (*Gan Cao*)   5 grams

Method of administration: Boil the last two herbs in 700ml of water for 15 minutes. Add the green Tea, and bring back to a boil. Then remove from the heat. Discard the dregs, save the liquid, and drink warm. Use 1 packet per day taken in 3 doses.

Functions: Cools and quickens the blood, dispels stasis and combats cancer

Indications: This tea is suitable for the treatment of leukemia exhibiting a pattern of blood heat and blood stasis. The blood stasis is typically evidenced by the easy bruising with so-called black and blue marks.

Sugar Added Flavors Red Date Tea (*Tang Jian Jia Wei Hong Zao Cha*)

Red dates, *i.e.*, Fructus Zizyphi Jujubae (*Da Zao*)	50 grams
Brown sugar (*Hong Tang*)	50 grams
Shelled raw peanuts (*Hua Sheng Mi*)	100 grams

Method of administration: Steep the red dates in warm water. Boil the peanuts slightly and let them cool. Remove the skin from the peanuts. Place the steeped red dates and peanut skins into the water which was used to boil the peanuts. Add a suitable amount of cold water and boil over a gentle fire for 1/2 hour. Remove the peanut skins and add the brown sugar. When the sugar has dissolved, use this liquid. Drink it warm as a tea, using 1 packet per day.

Functions: Supplements and engenders the blood

Indications: This tea is suitable for the treatment of leukemia and cancer patients with anemia after radiation therapy and chemotherapy as evidenced by a pale facial complexion, pale lips and nails, fatigue, and night sweats.

14
Miscellaneous Diseases

Alcohol Toxin Teas

Alcohol toxins are due to excessive drinking of alcohol which causes smoldering of dampness and brewing of heat internally. Thus wine toxins accumulate. The symptoms of this condition are a red face and eyes, vexatious heat and stirring agitation, a burning sensation in the region of the heart, hiccough and nausea, a desire to vomit all the time, uncontrollable speech, abnormal crying or laughing, and a drunken, clouded spirit In the worst cases, alcohol toxins may cause death. "Drinker's jaundice," a disease category recorded in ancient Chinese books, belongs to the category of alcohol toxins in the more modern TCM literature. Tea formulas have fairly good results for resolving alcohol toxins as long as the person does not continue drinking alcohol. In other words, as far back as Li Dong-yuan in his *Pi Wei Lun (Treatise on the Spleen & Stomach)*, Chinese herbal medicines for the treatment of the ill effects of alcohol intoxication should not be considered a *carte blanche* to continue drinking.

White Vinegar Resolve Alcohol Tea (*Bai Cu Jie Jiu Cha*)

White vinegar (*Bai Cu*)   10ml
White sugar (*Bai Tang*)   Amount to taste

Method of administration: Pour the white vinegar into a cup, add 50ml of boiling water, and then add white sugar. Drink slowly.

Functions: Dispels the effects of alcohol, increases the appetite or opens the stomach, and resolves toxins

Indications: This tea is suitable for the treatment of poor appetite and excessive drinking of alcohol.

Orange Peel Resolve Alcohol Tea (*Gan Pi Jie Jiu Cha*)

Orange peel dried over a fire (*Gan Zi Pi*)	60 grams
Tea leaves, *i.e.,* Folium Camelliae Theae (*Cha Ye*)	Small amount

Method of administration: Boil the orange peel 3-5 times and then add the Tea leaves. Drink immediately.

Functions: Dispels the effects of alcohol, transforms dampness, and increases the appetite.

Indications: This tea can be used to treat the effects of excessive consumption of alcohol as well as poor appetite.

Summerheat Stroke Teas

Summerheat stroke is an acute and dangerous condition due to exposure to excessively high temperatures for a period of time, for instance while working under the scorching hot sun. Its symptoms are characterized by a high body temperature (105° F or higher), headache, dizziness, numbness, and the cessation of sweating. If severe, there may be symptoms of confusion, sudden fainting, uneven or rapid breathing, and a fast pulse. Because this condition can be life-threatening, treatment should utilize Western medical emergency methods, as well as TCM. The focus of the formulas below is on the prevention of this condition.

Summerheat Prevention Tea (*Fang Shu Cha*)

Tea leaves, *i.e.*, Folium Camelliae Theae (*Cha Ye*)	6 grams
Herba Agastachis Seu Pogostemi (*Huo Xiang*)	9 grams
Herba Eupatorii Fortunei (*Pei Lan*)	9 grams

Method of administration: Rinse the last two ingredients well. Place the herbs in a cup with the Tea leaves and pour boiling water into the cup.
Functions: Clears heat and resolves summerheat

Indications: This tea is suitable for the treatment of light summerheat stroke.

Cooling Watermelon Peel Tea (*Cui Yi Liang Cha*)

Fresh watermelon peel, *i.e.*, fresh Exocarpium Citrulli Vulgaris (*Xian Xi Gua Pi*)	9 grams
Stir-fried gardenia fruit, *i.e.*, stir-fried Fructus Gardenia Jasminoidis (*Chao Zhi Zi*)	3.6 grams
Red peony root, *i.e.*, Radix Rubrus Paeoniae Lactiflorae (*Chi Shao*)	6 grams
Rhizoma Coptidis Chinensis (*Huang Lian*)	1 gram
Licorice root, *i.e.*, Radix Glycyrrhizae Uralensis (*Gan Cao*)	1 gram
White sugar (*Bai Tang*)	10 grams

Method of administration: Chop the watermelon peel into small cubes and place them in a pot with the other herbs. Add 1 ½ bowls of water and simmer for 20 minutes. Discard the dregs and keep the liquid. Add the sugar to the liquid, stir, and drink when cool. Use 1 packet per day.

Functions: Clears summerheat and disinhibits water

Indications: This tea is mainly used for summerheat stroke with fever, vexation and agitation, thirst, and short voidings of yellow urine.

Clear Summerheat & Brighten the Eyes Tea (*Qing Shu Ming Mu Cha*)

White chrysanthemum flower, *i.e.*, Flos Chrysanthemi Morifolii (*Bai Ju Hua*)	10 grams
Semen Cassiae Torae (*Jue Ming Zi*)	10 grams
Flos Immaturus Sophorae Japonicae (*Huai Hua Mi*)	10 grams

Method of administration: Boil these three ingredients in water. Drink when cool.

Functions: Clears heat and dispels summerheat, calms the liver and lowers pressure

Indications: This tea is suitable for a heavy head with dizzy vision due to summerheat and hypertension.

Lophatherum & Licorice Clear the Heart Tea (*Zhu Gan Qing Xin Cha*)

Herba Lophatheri Gracilis (*Dan Zhu Ye*)	15 grams
Licorice root, *i.e.*, Radix Glycyrrhizae Uralensis (*Gan Cao*)	10 grams
Field mint or peppermint, *i.e.*, Herba Menthae Haplocalycis (*Bo He*)	3 grams
White sugar (*Bai Tang*)	Amount to taste

Method of administration: Boil the lophatherum and licorice with 800ml water in a pot for 10 minutes. Add the mint and return to a brief boil. Discard the dregs and retain the liquid. When cool, add the sugar. Take 1 packet per day.

Functions: Clears heat and resolves vexation, clears summerheat and dispels dampness

Indications: This tea is suitable for summerheat, thirst, vexation, and reddish yellow urination. In China, it is a common cooling drink for the summertime.

Daqingye & Honeysuckle Tea (*Da Qing Yin Hua Cha*)

Fresh Folium Daqingye (*Xian Da Qing Ye*)   30-60 grams
Honeysuckle flower, *i.e.*, Flos Lonicerae Japonicae (*Jin Yin Hua*) 15-30 grams
Tea leaves, *i.e.*, Folium Camelliae Theae (*Cha Ye*)   5 grams

Note: If the Folium Daqingye is dry, use only 20 grams.

Method of administration: Either boil the three ingredients with water or soak them in boiling water for 20 minutes. Take 1 packet per day at any time.

Functions: Clears heat, resolves toxins, and dispels summerheat

Indications: This tea is suitable for the treatment of epidemic encephalitis B and summerheat stroke with high fever. It can also be drunk preventively against summerheat and infection.

Mint & Elsholtzia (*Bo He Xiang Cha*)

Field mint or peppermint, *i.e.*, Herba Menthae Haplocalycis (*Bo He*) 4 grams
Herba Elsholtziae Splendentis (*Xiang Ru*)   3 grams
Herba Lophatheri Gracilis (*Dan Zhu Ye*)   3 grams
Plantain leaves, *i.e.*, Herba Plantaginis (*Qian He Cao* or *Che Qian Cao*) 5 grams

Method of administration: Rinse the elsholtzia, lophatherum, and plantain well. Boil them with water in a pot for 5 minutes. Then add the mint and boil for another 5 minutes. Take 1 packet per day.

Functions: Disperses summerheat and clears heat

Indications: This tea is suitable for the prevention of summerheat and the treatment of symptoms such as chest oppression, vexation, thirst, and short voidings of reddish urine due to summerheat. It is a good tea for protection from heat.

Lotus Leaf & Stem Tea (*He Ye Lian Gen Cha*)

Folium Nelumbinis Nuciferae (*He Ye*)   10 grams
Ramulus Nelumbinis Nuciferae (*Lian Gen*)   15 grams

Method of administration: Rinse the lotus leaves and stems well, tear into pieces, and steep in boiling water. Take 1 packet per day.
Functions: Disperses summerheat and loosens the chest, engenders fluids and stops thirst, frees the qi and relaxes the sinews

Indications: This tea is suitable for the prevention of summerheat. If taken often, symptoms such as vexation, thirst, chest and diaphragmatic oppression and distention due to damp heat can be eliminated.

15
Teas for TCM Patterns

Bodily Vacuity & Qi Weakness Teas

Bodily vacuity and qi weakness mainly refers to qi vacuity. In TCM, qi vacuity is usually due to vacuity and detriment of one or more of the viscera and bowels, such as lung qi vacuity and/or spleen qi vacuity. It may also be due to severe illness or chronic disease reducing and consuming the original qi. General symptoms are a drained, white facial complexion, dizziness, tinnitus, heart palpitations, shortness of breath, sweating on slight exertion, a low and faint voice, and fatigue. The medicinal teas given below all help to support and assist the righteous qi and strengthen the body's ability to resist externally invading disease.

Ginseng Tea (*Ren Shen Cha*)

White ginseng, *i.e.*, white Radix Panacis Ginseng (*Bai Ren Shen*)   8 grams

Method of administration: Boil the ginseng 3 times, filter it, and add a suitable amount of boiled water to the liquid. Drink this as a tea, 1 packet per day.

Functions: Greatly supplements the original qi, supplements the spleen and boosts the lungs, engenders fluid and secures desertion, quiets the spirit and boosts the brain

Indications: This tea is suitable for the treatment of chronic illness with qi vacuity, spleen and lung insufficiency, poor appetite, shortness of breath, spontaneous sweating, fatigue, a yellowish white facial complexion with little luster, a vacuous pulse, fluid injury, oral thirst, thirsting and wasting, insomnia, and/or heart palpitations.

Contraindications: This formula should not be taken at the same time with radish or Tea. It is contraindicated for individuals with yin vacuity and fire effulgence.

Ginseng & Fruit Juice Tea (*Ren Shen Guo Lu Cha*)

Ginseng, *i.e.*, Radix Panacis Ginseng (*Ren Shen*)	10 grams
Pineapple juice (*Bo Luo Zhi*)	30 grams
White sugar (*Bai Tang*)	50 grams
Honey (*Feng Mi*)	60 grams

Method of administration: Wash the ginseng well, cut it into thin slices, steep with hot water, and then pound into pieces. Add a small amount of white sugar to macerate. Heat the rest of the sugar and the honey in 500ml of water and bring to a boil. Add the pineapple juice and stir well. Then add the ginseng juice and stir again. Use 2 spoonfuls of the juice for each dose. Pour hot water over the juice in a cup and drink it as a tea 2-3 times a day.

Functions: Greatly supplements the original qi

Indications: This tea is suitable for the treatment of lassitude of the spirit, lack of strength, shortness of breath, spontaneous perspiration, and a clouded head with impaired memory. It can enhance cerebral cortex function, increase one's ability to work, reduce fatigue, and strengthen the organic body's immune system. It can also regulate cholesterol and metabolism and improve digestive and absorption functions. It facilitates protein synthesis and is one of the best drinks to take in winter.

Contraindications: This tea should not be taken at the same time with radish and/or Tea. Individuals with yin vacuity and fire effulgence should not drink this tea.

Astragalus Tea (*Huang Qi Cha*)

Uncooked Radix Astragali Membranacei (*Sheng Huang Qi*)   60-90 grams
Red dates, *i.e.*, Fructus Zizyphi Jujubae (*Da Zao*)   30 grams

Method of administration: Boil these two ingredients with water for 30 minutes and then drink. Use 1 packet per day. The same herb packet can be boiled repeatedly. According to the disease condition, this formula can be taken continuously for 1 week to 3 months.

Functions: Supplements the qi and upbears yang, secures the exterior and stops sweating, fortifies the spleen and nourishes the blood

Indications: This tea is suitable for the treatment of a lusterless facial complexion, fatigue, shortness of breath, and spontaneous perspiration. Taken often, this tea is very strengthening.

Ginseng Root-neck Tea (*Shen Lu Cha*)

Ginseng root-neck, *i.e.*, Cervix Radicis Panacis Ginseng (*Ren Shen Lu*)   5 grams
Crystal sugar (*Bing Tang*)   Amount to taste

Method of administration: Steep the ginseng root-neck in boiling water for 30 minutes. It is best to cut it into thin slices first. An alternate method is to add water and crystal sugar to the ginseng root-neck and boil separately with water for 30 minutes. Drink 1 packet every 2 days. This formula can be steeped for 3-4 times and drunk warm at any time as a tea.

Functions: Supplements the qi and strengthens the kidneys, fortifies the spleen and boosts the lungs, dispels disease and prolongs life

Indications: This tea is suitable for the treatment of qi vacuity, kidney depletion, fatigue, low back pain, and susceptibility to catching cold as well as all male and female vacuity symptoms. This tea may also be used as an adjunctive treatment for cancer if the patient exhibits a pronounced qi vacuity pattern of signs and symptoms or a qi and blood vacuity pattern.

Pseudostellaria & Wheat Tea (*Shen Mai Cha*)

Radix Pseudostellariae Heterophyllae (*Tai Zi Shen*)   9 grams
Blighted wheat, *i.e.*, Semen Levis Tritici Aestivi (*Fu Xiao Mai*)   15 grams

Method of administration: Place these two herbs in a thermos and steep in boiling water for 20 minutes. Drink this as a tea, 1 packet per day.

Functions: Boosts the qi and constrains sweating

Indications: This tea is suitable for the treatment of qi and blood insufficiency or depletion and vacuity after illness. It may also be used for symptoms of constant spontaneous perspiration, no pleasure in eating, fatigue, heart palpitations, and a dry mouth.

Yin Blood Depletion & Detriment Teas

Yin blood depletion and detriment is also called constructive and blood depletion and detriment. It includes liver blood insufficiency and heart/spleen vacuity diseases. Its symptoms are a pale or sallow yellow facial complexion, dizziness, vertigo, flusteredness, shortness of breath, light purple lips and tongue, scanty menstruation, delayed menstruation, or blocked menstruation, *i.e.*, amenorrhea. This pattern is often seen in different kinds of anemia, hematological diseases, and cancer as well as different kinds of chronic vacuity diseases.

Longan Tea (*Long Yan Cha*)

Longan fruit, *i.e.*, Arillus Euphoriae Longanae (*Long Yan Rou*)   5-10 pieces

Method of administration: Place this herb in a double boiler and steam thoroughly. Remove and then place in a teacup. Steep in boiling water, remove the dregs, and drink as a tea, 1 packet per day.

Functions: Boosts the heart and spleen, supplements the qi and blood, and quiets the spirit

Indications: This tea is suitable for the treatment of a weak constitution, blood vacuity, neurasthenia, fright palpitations, impaired memory, and insomnia due to heart blood vacuity.

Lycium & Schisandra Tea (*Gou Qi Wu Wei Cha*)

Fructus Lycii Chinensis (*Gou Qi Zi*)	Equal amount
Fructus Schisandrae Chinensis (*Wu Wei Zi*)	Equal amount

Method of administration: Grind these two ingredients into a coarse powder. Twice a day, steep 5 grams of this powder in boiling water and drink as a tea. The herbs may also be eaten.

Functions: Enriches and supplements the essence and blood

Indications: This tea is suitable for the treatment of essence/blood insufficiency, dizziness, tinnitus, heart palpitations, insomnia, cloudy vision, seminal emission, and chronic hepatitis.

Red Dates Nourish the Blood Tea (*Hong Zao Yang Xue Cha*)

Red dates, *i.e.*, Fructus Zizyphus Jujubae (*Hong Zao*)	10 pieces
Green Tea, *i.e.*, Folium Camelliae Theae (*Lu Cha*)	5 grams
White sugar (*Bai Tang*)	10 grams

Method of administration: Boil the red dates in water with the white sugar until the red dates are thoroughly cooked. Steep the green Tea in boiling water for 5 minutes and then pour the Tea water into the red dates soup. Stir evenly and drink warm. Use 1 packet per day taken at any time.

Functions: Supplements the essence and nourishes the blood, fortifies the spleen and harmonizes the stomach

Indications: This tea is suitable for the treatment of chronic illness, bodily vacuity, anemia, and vitamin deficiency.

Polygonum Tea (*He Shou Wu Cha*)

Radix Polygoni Multiflori (*He Shou Wu*)   6 grams

Method of administration: Cut the herb into thin slices and steep in boiling water. Drink the same tea packet until the flavor has become weak, 1-2 times per day.

Functions: Supplements the liver and boosts the kidneys, nourishes the blood and dispels wind

Indications: This tea is suitable for the treatment of yin vacuity and blood dryness, premature graying of the hair, weak sinews and bones, and insomnia. This formula is good for enriching and supplementing the elderly with weak constitutions and individuals with anemia. It may be taken often by such persons.

Dang Gui Supplement the Blood Tea (*Dang Gui Bu Xue Cha*)

Radix Angelicae Sinensis (*Dang Gui*)   10 grams
Prepared Radix Rehmanniae (*Shu Di*)   10 grams
Red dates, *i.e.*, Fructus Ziziphi Jujubae (*Da Zao*)   30 grams

Method of administration: Place the above herbs into a pot with water and boil. Use 1 packet per day. Drink this at any time as a tea.

Functions: Nourishes and supplements the blood

Indications: This tea is suitable for the treatment of yin and blood depletion and vacuity with symptoms such as a weak body, a sallow yellow facial complexion, and menstrual irregularity in females.

268

Salvia & Polygonatum Tea (*Dan Shen Huang Jing Cha*)

Radix Salviae Miltiorrhizae (*Dan Shen*)	10 grams
Rhizoma Polygonati (*Huang Jing*)	10 grams
Green Tea, *i.e.*, Folium Camelliae Theae (*Lu Cha*)	5 grams

Method of administration: Grind the above ingredients into a coarse powder, steep in boiling water, cover for 10 minutes, and then drink. Use 1 packet per day.

Functions: Quickens and supplements the blood, replenishes the essence

Indications: This tea is suitable for the treatment of anemia and leukopenia.

Qi & Yin Dual Vacuity Teas

Qi and yin dual vacuity, also called qi and yin damage, refers to the consumption and damage of both yin fluids and yang qi. It usually occurs as a result of heat disease or chronic, wasting diseases. If the condition is relatively light, it is called qi and yin insufficiency. If it is relatively severe, it is called qi and yin vacuity. Its symptoms are low-grade fever, sensations of heat in the hands and feet, spontaneous perspiration, night sweats, lassitude of the spirit, fatigue, shortness of breath, disinclination to speak, oral thirst, a dry mouth and dry throat, a red tongue with little or no coating, and a deep, fine, rapid, and vacuous pulse. This pattern is usually seen after a high fever or surgery. It is also seen in Western medical diseases such as pulmonary tuberculosis and diabetes.

American Ginseng Tea (*Xi Yang Shen Cha*)

American ginseng, *i.e.*, Radix Panacis Quinquefolii (*Xi Yang Shen*)	1-2 grams

Method of administration: Cut this herb into thin slices and steep in boiling water for 20 minutes. This tea may be taken once a day at any time.

Functions: Boosts the qi and engenders fluids, moistens the lungs and clears heat

Indications: This tea is suitable for the treatment of qi and yin vacuity which causes shortness of breath, lack of strength, and dry mouth. It is also useful for lung and stomach yin vacuity, a low-grade fever, or vacuity fire flaming upward with mouth and tongue sores.

Ginseng Rootlets Tea (*Ren Shen Xu Cha*)

Ginseng rootlets, *i.e.*, rootlets of Radix Panacis Ginseng (*Ren Shen Xu*)	3 grams
Umeboshi, *i.e.*, Fructus Pruni Mume (*Wu Mei*)	6 grams
White sugar (*Bai Tang*)	Amount to taste

Method of administration: Steep the above herbs in boiling water. Drink this often as a tea.

Functions: Supplements vacuity and strengthens the body, engenders fluids and stops thirst

Indications: This tea is suitable for the treatment of thirst, spontaneous perspiration, shortness of breath, and lack of strength. It is also suitable for summerheat damaging the fluids and consuming the qi.

Codonopsis & Ophiopogon Tea (*Dang Shen Mai Dong Cha*)

Radix Codonopsitis Pilosulae (*Dang Shen*)	25 grams
Tuber Ophiopogonis Japonici (*Mai Men Dong*)	10 grams
Fructus Schisandrae Chinensis (*Wu Wei Zi*)	6 grams
Red dates, *i.e.*, Fructus Zizyphi Jujubae (*Da Zao*)	50 grams
Crystal sugar (*Bing Tang*)	Amount to taste

Method of administration: Place these four herbs into a pot, add 1,000ml of water, boil until 800ml of liquid remain. Add the crystal sugar, allow it to dissolve, and stir well. Use 1 packet per day split into several doses throughout the day.

Functions: Boosts the qi and nourishes yin, fortifies the spleen and increases the appetite

Indications: This tea is suitable for the treatment of qi and yin insufficiency, low spirit, shortness of breath, disinclination to speak, fatigue, and chronic cough with scant phlegm as well as a weak constitution.

Engender the Pulse Tea (*Sheng Mai Cha*)

Ginseng, *i.e.*, Radix Panacis Ginseng (*Ren Shen*) — 9 grams
Tuber Ophiopogonis Japonici (*Mai Men Dong*) — 15 grams
Fructus Schisandrae Chinensis (*Wu Wei Zi*) — 6 grams

Method of administration: Boil the above herbs with water. Drink the resulting liquid repeatedly as a tea.

Functions: Boosts the qi and nourishes yin, constrains perspiration and engenders the pulse

Indications: This tea is suitable for the treatment of qi and yin decline, copious perspiration, and a very faint pulse. It may also be used for a weak constitution with low blood pressure, dizziness, lack of strength, shortness of breath, a dry mouth, red tongue, and a soft, vacuous pulse. In addition, it treats summerheat damage with symptoms of copious perspiration, thirst due to damaged fluids and consumed qi, lassitude of the spirit, a dry tongue with red color, and a vacuous, weak, forceless pulse.

Pseudostellaria & Dendrobium Tea (*Shen Hu Cha*)

Radix Pseudostellariae Heterophyllae (*Tai Zi Shen*) — 15 grams
Herba Dendrobii (*Shi Hu*) — 10 grams
Fructus Schisandrae Chinensis (*Wu Wei Zi*) — 6 pieces

271

Method of administration: Chop the above herbs into pieces and then grind them into a fine powder. Place in a container and steep with boiling water. Drink as a tea once a day.

Functions: Boosts the qi and nourishes yin, clears heat and engenders fluids

Indications: This tea is suitable for the treatment of heat disease that has damaged yin with one symptom being a dry mouth with thirst. It also treats stomach yin insufficiency with symptoms of abdominal pain and dry heaves. The tongue is smooth with little or no coating. It may also be used in the elderly with shortness of breath, lack of strength, dizziness, and heart palpitations.

Sweet Chrysanthemum Tea (*Tian Ju Cha*)

Sweet chrysanthemum flower, *i.e.*, sweet Flos Chrysanthemi
    Morifolii (*Tian Ju Hua*)   6-9 grams

Method of administration: Steep this herb in boiling water for 5 minutes and then drink. Use 1 packet per day at any time.

Functions: Nourishes yin and engenders fluids

Indications: This tea is suitable for the treatment of stomach yin insufficiency and dry mouth with thirst. It is also useful for hypertension, diabetes, obesity, or for patients who need to control their sugar intake.

Butter Tea (*Su You Cha*)

Butter (*Huang You*)	150 grams
Brick Tea (*Zuan Cha*)	Amount to taste
Table salt (*Jing Yan*)	Amount to taste
Cow's milk (*Niu Nai*)	1 cup

Method of administration: Place 100 grams of butter, 5 grams of table salt, and the milk into a clean container. Into the same container, pour in about 400-800ml of pre-made Tea water. Use a clean, thin wooden spatula to beat for 5 minutes. Then add the last 50 grams of butter and beat for another 2 minutes. After the second beating, pour the mixture into a teapot and heat briefly, up to 1 minute. It should not be boiled because the tea and butter will separate and the taste will be unpleasant. Drink this at any time.

Functions: Enriches yin and supplements the qi, fortifies the spleen and lifts the spirit

Indications: This tea is suitable for treatment after an illness or postpartum as well as for different types of weak individuals. It enhances the constitution, increases the appetite, and speeds recovery.

Yang Qi Insufficiency Teas

Yang qi insufficiency means yang vacuity. Its clinical symptoms are a drained or somber white facial complexion, cold hands and feet, easy perspiration, loose stools, clear, long urine, pale lips, and a bland taste in the mouth. The tongue is pale in color, moist, and has a white coating. The pulse is vacuous and weak. The following tea formulas can be chosen depending on the individual person's symptoms.

Codonopsis & Stir-fried Rice Tea (*Dang Shen Chao Mi Cha*)

Radix Codonopsitis Pilosulae (*Dang Shen*)	15-30 grams
Stir-fried rice (*Chao Mi*)	30 grams

Method of administration: Place these two ingredients in a pot and add 4 bowls of water. Boil until 1 1/2 bowls of water are left. Drink this as a tea, once every other day.

Functions: Warms yang and boosts the qi, fortifies the spleen and harmonizes the stomach

Indications: This tea is suitable for the treatment of spleen yang vacuity with symptoms of decreased appetite, fatigue, cold body and limbs, watery diarrhea or undigested food in the stools, rumbling intestines with abdominal pain, and white or watery vaginal discharge. The tongue is pale with a white coating. The pulse is vacuous and weak or deep and slow.

Contraindications: Do not use this tea in individuals with yin vacuity fire effulgence or who are strong and in robust health. It is also not suitable to take this tea during the hottest part of the summer. Autumn and winter are the most appropriate seasons to use it.

Codonopsis & Red Date Tea (*Dang Shen Hong Zao Cha*)

Radix Codonopsitis Pilosulae (*Dang Shen*)   15-30 grams
Red dates, *i.e.*, Fructus Zizyphi Jujubae (*Hong Zao*)   5-10 pieces

Note: If available, one can substitute black dates (*Hei Zao*) for the red dates. These are red dates which have been prepared specially to make them warmer and more supplementing to the yang qi. In their processing, their color turns from red to black and hence their Chinese name. *Hong Zao* and *Da Zao* both refer to red dates.

Method of administration: Boil these two ingredients in water. Drink the resulting liquid as a tea, using 1 packet per day.

Functions: Warms yang and boosts the qi

Indications: This tea is suitable for the treatment of heart yang vacuity with symptoms of heart palpitations, spontaneous perspiraton, fatigue, shortness of breath, somnolence, cold body and limbs, stifling oppression in the heart and chest, and a pale, white facial complexion. The tongue is either pale or dark purple. The pulse is thin and weak or bound and regularly interrupted.

274

Qi & Blood Dual Vacuity Teas

Dual vacuity of the qi and blood refers to both qi vacuity and blood vacuity manifesting at the same time. Thus there are signs of qi vacuity, such as fatigued essence-spirit, lack of strength, disinclination to speak, spontaneous perspiration, and decreased appetite, as well as the symptoms of blood vacuity, such as a sallow yellow facial complexion, heart palpitations, racing of the heart, vertigo, tinnitus, and dry, withered nails. This dual vacuity is usually due to chronic illness or great blood loss. It can be seen in many types of chronic diseases and different types of anemia, as well as in postpartum blood vacuity. The following tea formulas can be useful in treatment.

Cow's Milk & Black Tea (*Niu Ru Hong Cha*)

Cow's milk (*Niu Nai*)   100 grams
Black Tea, *i.e.*, prepared Folium Camelliae Theae (*Hong Cha*)   Amount to taste
Table salt (*Jing Yan*)   Amount to taste

Method of administration: Boil the black Tea with water and dispose of the dregs. Boil the cow's milk. Mix the boiled milk and thick black Tea water together, adding a small amount of table salt. Drink this once a day in the morning on an empty stomach.

Functions: Enriches and nourishes the qi and blood, supplements the liver and strengthens the body

Indications: This tea is suitable for the treatment of qi and blood insufficiency, such as postpartum and after a debilitating illness.

Nourish the Blood Tea (*Yang Xue Cha*)

Red dates, *i.e.*, Fructus Zizyphi Jujubae (*Da Zao*)   50 grams
Uncooked ginger, *i.e.*, Rhizoma Zingiberis (*Sheng Jiang*)   5 grams
Brown sugar (*Hong Tang*)   Amount to taste

Method of administration: Wash the ginger and cut it into slices. Place the ginger and red dates into a pot, add a suitable amount of water, and bring to a boil. Boil over a gentle fire for 20 minutes. Add the brown sugar and stir evenly. Drink this while warm.

Functions: Boosts the qi and nourishes the blood

Indications: This tea is suitable for the treatment of qi and blood insufficiency with symptoms of a yellow facial complexion, heart palpitations, racing of the heart, shortness of breath, and lack of strength. It is also suitable for spleen and stomach vacuity and coldness.

Longan & Crystal Sugar Tea (*Long Yan Bing Tang Cha*)

Longan fruit, *i.e.*, Arillus Euphoriae Longanae (*Long Yan Rou*)   10 grams
Crystal sugar (*Bing Tang*)   3 grams

Method of administration: Place the longan fruit and sugar together in a teacup. Pour in boiling water and steep. Drink this as a tea. One can repeatedly steep the fruit by adding more boiled water.

Functions: Supplements the heart and spleen and boosts the qi and blood

Indications: This tea is suitable for the treatment of anemia, insomnia, heart palpitations, and profuse dreams.

Contraindications: Persons who have not yet recovered completely from an acute cold and individuals with poor digestion should not drink this tea.

Longan & American Ginseng Tea (*Long Yan Yang Shen Cha*)

Longan fruit, *i.e.*, Arillus Euphoriae Longanae (*Long Yan Rou*)   30 grams
American ginseng, *i.e.*, Radix Panacis Quinquefolii (*Xi Yang Shen*)   6 grams
White sugar (*Bai Tang*)   Amount to taste

Method of administration: Soak and moisten the American ginseng in water in order to soften it. Then cut it into slices. Clean and wash the longan fruit. Place these two herbs, white sugar, and a suitable amount of water into a double boiler and steam for 40-50 minutes. Take this tea in the morning and evening. One may also eat the herbs in addition to drinking the medicinal tea.

Functions: Boosts the qi and nourishes the blood, tranquilizes the heart and quiets the spirit

Indications: This tea is suitable for the treatment of heart palpitations, shortness of breath, insomnia, and impaired memory.

Kuan Yin's Personal Tea (*Guan Yin Mian Cha*)

Black sesame seed, *i.e.*, black Semen Sesami Indici (*Hei Zhi Ma*)	500 grams
Lotus root starch (*Ou Fen*)	500 grams
Polished, round-grained, non-glutinous rice, *i.e.*, Semen Oryzae Sativae (*Jing Mi*)	500 grams
White sugar (*Bai Tang*)	500 grams
Radix Dioscoreae Oppositae (*Shan Yao*)	500 grams

Method of administration: Stir-fry the sesame, rice, and dioscorea until they are cooked. Grind them into a fine powder. Sift this powder and use the very finest part. Mix this fine powder with the lotus root starch and white sugar and store it in a sealed container. To use, place 30 grams in a container, pour in hot water, stir evenly, and drink. This tea may be used as a breakfast or snack food.

Functions: Boosts the qi and blood, blackens the hair and beard, and helps to retard aging

Indications: This tea is suitable for the treatment of qi and blood vacuity with symptoms of premature graying of the hair and premature senility.

Note: The name of this tea has a double meaning in Chinese. The word *mian* means face, personal, and a fine flour.

Eight Immortals Tea (*Ba Xian Cha*)

Polished, round-grained, non-glutinous rice, *i.e.*, Semen Oryzae Sativae (*Jing Mi*)	750 grams
Millet (*Su Mi*)	750 grams
Soybean, *i.e.*, Semen Glycinis (*Huang Dou*)	750 grams
Aduki bean, *i.e.*, Semen Phaseoli Calcarati (*Chi Xiao Dou*)	750 grams
Mung bean, *i.e.*, Semen Phaseoli Munginis (*Lu Dou*)	750 grams

(Stir-fry the above five ingredients until they are well cooked.)

Fine Tea, *i.e.*, fine Folium Camelliae Theae (*Xi Cha*)	500 grams
Sesame seed, *i.e.*, Semen Sesami Indici (*Zhi Ma*)	375 grams
Szechuan pepper, *i.e.,* Pericarpium Zanthoxyli Bungeani (*Hua Jiao*)	75 grams
Fennel seed, *i.e.*, Fructus Foeniculi Vulgaris (*Xiao Hui Xiang*)	150 grams
Blast-fried, dry ginger, *i.e.*, blast-fried, dry Rhizoma Zingiberis (*Pao Gan Jiang*)	30 grams

(Roast the above five ingredients in a pan.)

Stir-fried salt crystal (*Chao Jing Yan*)	30 grams

Method of administration: Grind the above 11 ingredients into a fine powder and mix. Stir-fry a suitable amount of wheat flour until it is yellow and cooked. Then mix this with the other 11 kinds of powder. Store in a sealed container. When using, walnuts, pinenuts, and white sugar may be added to individual taste. Three times a day, use 3 spoonfuls of the above powder or 6-9 grams. Steep in boiling water and drink the resulting liquid warm. This powder may also be swallowed and chased with hot water.

Functions: Supplements the essence and moistens the skin, safeguards the original qi and secures the kidneys

278

Indications: This tea is suitable for the treatment of qi and blood insufficiency with symptoms of fatigue, easily catching cold, fear of the cold, chilling of the four limbs, and dry, rough skin. It is also useful for debilitation of the life-gate fire and kidney qi insufficiency.

Spleen & Stomach Vacuity Teas

The spleen and stomach are the earth viscus. They are the root of postnatal or latter heaven qi and blood engenderment and transformation. Common symptoms of spleen/stomach vacuity are a sallow yellow facial complexion, fatigue, weak essence-spirit, weakness of the four limbs, shortness of breath, disinclination to speak, decreased appetite, epigastric and abdominal pain, glomus and fullness in the epigastrium and abdomen, loose stools, and diarrhea. The tongue is pale with thin, white coating. The pulse is fine and weak. The following formulas have the effect of supplementing and boosting the spleen and stomach and can be chosen for different conditions.

Poria & Cow's Milk Tea (*Fu Ling Nai Cha*)

Powdered Sclerotium Poriae Cocos (*Fu Ling Fen*)	10 grams
Cow's milk (*Niu Nai*)	200mls

Method of administration: Use a small amount of cool, boiled water to dissolve the Poria. Then add the boiled cow's milk. Drink this tea in the morning on an empty stomach.

Functions: Fortifies the spleen and quiets the heart, enriches, supplements, and strengthens the body, retards aging

Indications: This tea is suitable for the treatment of spleen and stomach vacuity and poor digestion.

Fortify the Spleen Tea (*Jian Pi Cha*)

Rhizoma Atractylodis Macrocephalae (*Bai Zhu*)	20 grams
Radix Dioscoreae Oppositae (*Shan Yao*)	15 grams
Roasted kudzu root, *i.e.*, roasted Radix Puerariae (*Wei Ge Gen*)	9 grams
Tangerine peel, *i.e.*, Pericarpium Citri Reticulatae (*Chen Pi*)	6 grams

Method of administration: Boil the above four ingredients with water, remove the dregs, and drink. Use 1 packet per day.

Functions: Supplements and boosts the spleen and stomach

Indications: This tea is suitable for the treatment of spleen and stomach vacuity causing abdominal distention after meals, fatigue in the four limbs, and chronic diarrhea.

Codonopsis & Lycium Tea (*Shen Qi Cha*)

Radix Codonopsitis Pilosulae (*Dang Shen*)	9 grams
Fructus Lycii Chinensis (*Gou Qi Zi*)	6 grams

Method of administration: Boil these two herbs together and drink. Use 1 packet per day.

Functions: Boosts the qi, fortifies the spleen, and supplements the kidneys

Indications: This tea is suitable for the treatment of spleen and stomach vacuity, dual depletion of the qi and blood, and low back and knees soreness and weakness.

Clear Heat (Handed Down From the) Generations Tea Beverage (*Qing Re Dai Cha Yin*)

Fresh Rhizoma Phragmitis Communis (*Xian Lu Gen*)	2 stalks
Caulis Bambusae In Taeniis (*Zhu Ru*)	7.5 grams

Scorched hawthorn fruit, *i.e.*, scorched Fructus Crataegi
    (*Jiao Shan Zha*)   15 grams
Stir-fried germinated rice, *i.e.*, stir-fried Fructus Germinatus
    Oryzae Sativae (*Chao Gu Ya*)   15 grams
Red tangerine peel, *i.e.*, Exocarpium Citri Erythrocarpae (*Ju Hong*)   4 grams
Mulberry leaf, *i.e.*, Folium Mori Albi (*Sang Ye*)   10 grams

Method of administration: Boil the above herbs with water. Use 1 packet per day. Drink this as a tea.

Functions: Clears and disinhibits the head and eyes and regulates and harmonizes the spleen and stomach

Indications: This tea is suitable for the treatment of poor appetite, head distention and dizziness, and fatigue.

Lung Yin Vacuity & Detriment Teas

Lung yin vacuity is usually due to a prolonged illness or chronic pathogenic heat lodging in the lungs causing damage to lung yin. It may also be due to excessive perspiration which damages the yin of the lungs leaving the lung viscus unmoistened. Its main symptoms are a dry cough with scant phlegm or phlegm streaked with blood, shortness of breath, panting, and dry throat and mouth. In severe cases, there may be a low-grade fever in the afternoon, tidal fever, and night sweats. The tongue body is red with a dry coating, and the pulse is fine and rapid. The following tea formulas may be used for these symptoms.

White Wood Ear Tea (*Yin Er Cha*)

White wood ear, *i.e.*, Fructificatio Tremellae Fuciformis (*Yin Er*)   20 grams
Tea leaves, *i.e.*, Folium Camelliae Theae (*Cha Ye*)   5 grams
Crystal sugar (*Bing Tang*)   Amount to taste

Method of administration: Wash the white wood ears well. Place the herb, water, and crystal sugar in a pot and boil thoroughly. Steep the Tea leaves separately in boiling water for 5 minutes. Finally, pour the Tea water into the white wood ear tea and stir evenly. Use 1 packet per day. Drink at any time.

Functions: Enriches yin and downbears fire, moistens the lungs and stops cough

Indications: This tea is suitable for the treatment of yin vacuity cough, pulmonary tuberculosis, and low-grade fever.

Sesame Seed & Almond Tea (*Zhi Ma Xing Ren Cha*)

Black sesame seed, *i.e.*, black Semen Sesami Indici (*Hei Zhi Ma*)	10 grams
Almond (*Tian Xing Ren*)	8 grams
Crystal sugar (*Bing Tang*)	Amount to taste

Method of administration: Pound the sesame and almond together into pieces and then steep in boiling water. Add the crystal sugar to taste. This may be taken once or twice daily.

Functions: Moistens the lungs and stops coughing

Indications: This tea is suitable for the treatment of prolonged cough with scant phlegm that is due to lung yin insufficiency.

Adenophora Tea (*Sha Shen Cha*)

Radix Adenophorae Strictae (*Nan Sha Shen*)	15 grams

Method of administration: Boil the herb with water and drink the resulting liquid as a tea.

Functions: Nourishes yin and clears the lungs

Indications: This tea is suitable for the treatment of lung heat cough, cough with a red face, dry cough, and heart vexation.

Liver/Kidney Insufficiency Teas

The liver stores the blood, the kidneys store the essence, and essence and blood engender each other. Thus the liver and kidneys enrich and nourish each other. This means that chronic liver blood insufficiency and kidney essence depletion and detriment can cause liver and kidney yin vacuity. The clinical symptoms of this pattern are dizziness, tinnitus, lateral costal region pain, low back and knee soreness and weakness, a dry throat, red cheeks, night sweats, and vexatious heat in the five hearts. In men, symptoms may include seminal emission. In women, there may be menstrual irreguarity. The tongue is red with no coating, and the pulse is fine and rapid.

Sesame Nourish the Blood Tea (*Zhi Ma Yang Xue Cha*)

Black sesame seed, *i.e.*, black Semen Sesami Indici (*Hei Zhi Ma*)	6 grams
Tea leaves, *i.e.*, Folium Camelliae Theae (*Cha Ye*)	3 grams

Method of administration: Stir-fry the sesame seeds until yellow. Then boil the sesame seeds and Tea leaves together. An alternate method is to steep these two ingredients in boiling water in a lidded container for 10 minutes. Drink the herbal tea and eat the sesame seeds and the Tea leaves.

Functions: Enriches and supplements the liver and kidneys, nourishes the blood, and moistens the lungs

Indications: This tea is suitable for the treatment of liver and kidney depletion and vacuity, rough skin, brittle, yellow hair, possible premature greying of the hair, and tinnitus.

Reverse Age & Recover Vigor Tea (*Fan Lao Huan Tong Cha*)

Wu Long Tea, *i.e.*, Wu Long Folium Camelliae Theae (*Wu Long Cha*)	3 grams
Fructus Sophorae Japonicae (*Huai Jiao*)	18 grams
Chinese wax gourd peel, *i.e.*, Exocarpium Benincasae Hispidae (*Dong Gua Pi*)	18 grams
Hawthorn fruit, *i.e.*, Fructus Crataegi (*Shan Zha*)	15 grams
Radix Polygoni Multiflori (*He Shou Wu*)	30 grams

Method of administration: Boil the last four ingredients with clear water for 20 minutes. Remove the dregs and use the remaining liquid to make the Wu Long Tea. Use 1 packet per day, drunk warm.

Functions: Enriches and supplements the liver and kidneys, moistens and blackens the hair, disperses and reduces fat, prolongs and boosts life

Indications: This tea is suitable for the treatment of liver and kidney yin vacuity, dizziness, tinnitus, brittle, yellow hair, premature greying of the hair, obesity, hypertension, high cholesterol, and arteriosclerosis.

Polygonum & Pine Needle Tea (*Shou Wu Song Zhen Cha*)

Radix Polygoni Multiflori (*He Shou Wu*)	18 grams
Pine needles (*Song Zhen*)	30 grams
Wu Long Tea, *i.e.,* Wu Long Folium Camelliae Theae (*Wu Long Cha*)	5 grams

Method of administration: Boil the first two ingredients with clear water for 20 minutes and remove the dregs. Use this boiled medicinal liquid to make Wu Long Tea. Drink this after it steeps for 5 minutes. Use 1 packet per day.

Functions: Supplements essence and boosts the blood, supports the righteous and dispels evils

Indications: This tea is suitable for the treatment of liver/kidney depletion and vacuity. It is also useful for individuals who are engaged in chemical, radioactive, or agricultural chemical production, nuclear technology, or mining work. It may further be used for decreased white blood cell count following radiation and chemotherapy.

Lycium Enrich & Supplement Tea (*Gou Qi Zi Bu Cha*)

Fructus Lycii Chinensis (*Gou Qi Zi*)	10 grams
Fructus Schisandrae Chinensis (*Wu Wei Zi*)	6 grams

Method of administration: Grind these two herbs into a fine powder. Place this powder into a thermos, pour in 300ml of boiling water, and cover with the cup. Use 1 packet per day. Drink this repeatedly as a tea.

Functions: Enriches and supplements the liver and kidneys, nourishes the heart and constrains sweating, engenders liquids and stops thirst

Indications: This tea is suitable for the treatment of liver/kidney insufficiency, seminal emission, low back and knee soreness and weakness, thirst, insomnia, and dizziness.

Blacken the Hair Tea (*Wu Fa Cha*)

Radix Polygoni Multiflori (*He Shou Wu*)	15 grams
Uncooked Radix Rehmanniae (*Sheng Di*)	30 grams
Grain alcohol (*Bai Jiu*)	A suitable amount

Method of administration: Wash the two herbs with the alcohol and cut them into thin slices. Steep the herbs in boiling water. Drink this as a tea, using 1 packet for 3-6 days. Use continuously for 4 months.

Functions: Supplements the liver and kidneys, boosts the qi and blood, blackens the hair, and gives the face a pleasant color

Indications: This tea is suitable for the treatment of white hair in men between the ages of 30 and 50.

Loranthus Tea (*Sang Ji Sheng Cha*)

Dry Ramus Loranthi Seu Visci (*Gan Pin Sang Ji Sheng*)   15 grams

Method of administration: Boil the herb for 5-10 minutes. Drink the resulting liquid as a tea, 1 packet per day.

Functions: Supplements and boosts the liver and kidneys, strengthens and fortifies the sinews and bones

Indications: This tea is suitable for the treatment of liver/kidney insufficiency with low back and knee soreness and weakness, atrophy and weakness of the sinews and bones, foot qi, wind cold damp bi, uterine bleeding in pregnancy, and profuse uterine bleeding due to kidney vacuity.

Prolong the Years & Boost the Kidneys Tea (*Yan Nian Yi Shen Cha*)

Radix Polygoni Multiflori (*He Shou Wu*)   50 grams
Red dates, *i.e.*, Fructus Zizyphi Jujubae (*Da Zao*)   50 grams
Brown sugar (*Hong Tang*)   50 grams

Method of administration: Melt the brown sugar with a suitable amount of warm water and steep the two herbs in this sugar water for 1 week. Remove the herbs, dry, then repeat this process of steeping and drying until the sugar is all absorbed. Grind the herbs into a fine powder for use. Each time, pour boiling water over 10 grams of this powder. Drink warm.

Functions: Supplements the liver and boosts the kidneys, boosts the qi and nourishes the blood

Indications: This tea is suitable for the treatment of liver/kidney insufficiency with premature greying of the hair, blood vacuity, dizziness, low back and knee soreness and weakness, aching sinews and bones, seminal emission, and vaginal discharge. It is also suitable for stomach vacuity with little food intake and spleen weakness with loose stools.

Old Age Bodily Decline Teas

Bodily decline due to old age refers to that stage of life when the form, structure, and functions of the body begin to become weak and decrepit. Such changes due to aging include decreased immune response and increased rate of illness. In TCM, elderly individuals tend to show the symptoms of a dual qi and blood vacuity and insufficient energy. In order to combat this decline and debility due to aging and in addition to conserving one's health, cultivating a good emotional disposition, and getting regular physical exercise, medicinal teas taken regularly may be very beneficial for retarding aging.

Prevent Aging Tea (*Fang Lao Cha*)

Ganoderma Lucidum (*Ling Zhi*)	10 grams
Siberian ginseng, *i.e.*, Cortex Radicis Eleutherococci (*Ci Wu Jia*)	8 grams
Herba Epimedii (*Yin Yang Huo*)	6 grams

Method of administration: Place these three ingredients into a container, steep in boiling water, cover the container for 5 minutes, and then drink this as a tea. Use 1 packet per day.

Functions: Invigorates the sinews and bones and strengthens the heart

Indications: This tea is suitable for the treatment of early senility and impaired memory in the middle-aged. This tea formula is ideal for middle and old age. It strengthens the mind and fortifies the body. If taken often, this tea can prevent and cure illness, prolong life and boost longevity.

287

Siberian Ginseng Tea (*Ci Wu Jia Cha*)

Siberian ginseng, *i.e.*, Cortex Radicis Eleutherococci (*Ci Wu Jia*)   30 grams

Method of administration: Cut this herb into pieces and then grind into powder. Steep in boiling water. Use 1 packet per day. The same packet may be steeped repeatedly to make tea.

Functions: Regulates nervous system function and quiets the spirit, boosts the brain, *i.e.*, intelligence, and brightens the eyes. This tea also dispels wind and dampness and invigorates the sinews and bones, supplements the five viscera and increases physical strength, quickens the blood and transforms stasis.

Polygonatum Tea (*Huang Jing Cha*)

Rhizoma Polygonati (*Huang Jing*)   60 grams

Method of administration: Cut this herb into slices and steep in boiled water for about 10 minutes. Discard the dregs and then drink the liquid. Use 1 packet per day taken freely as a tea.

Functions: Fortifies the body, increases the memory, and blackens the hair

Indications: Modern scientific research has proven that this tea formula retards aging, fortifies the body, and promotes longevity. Taken often, it has the effect of enriching, supplementing, and strengthening the body. This tea is suitable for the treatment of the aged with symptoms of shortness of breath, lack of strength, slow movement, lassitude of the spirit and fatigue, and middle qi insufficiency.

Ganoderma Tea (*Ling Zhi Cha*)

Ganoderma Lucidum (*Ling Zhi*)   10 grams

Method of administration: Cut this herb into thin slices, steep in boiled water, and drink.

288

Functions: Supplements the middle and boosts the qi, benefits longevity and prolongs life

Indications: The herb treats deafness, disinhibits the joints, safeguards the spirit, boosts the essence and qi, hardens the sinews and bones, and improves the facial color. Taken often, this formula will prolong life and benefit longevity. It can also prevent and treat high cholesterol.

Arouse the Brain Tea (*Xing Nao Cha*)

Tuber Ophiopogonis Japonici (*Mai Men Dong*)	15 grams
Fructus Schisandrae Chinensis (*Wu Wei Zi*)	10 grams
Fructus Lycii Chinensis (*Gou Qi Zi*)	10 grams

Method of administration: Place these herbs in a container, pour in boiling water, and cover for 5 minutes. Drink the resulting liquid as a tea. Use 1-2 packets per day.

Functions: Enriches yin and moistens the lungs, supplements the kidneys and nourishes the heart

Indications: This tea is suitable for the treatment of old age with body decline and decreased memory, dizziness, copious sweating, heart vexation in the summer, and a dry mouth and tongue. Taken often, this formula can arouse the brain and brighten the eyes, benefit longevity and prolong life.

Protect the Health Tea (*Bao Jian Cha*)

Radix Salviae Miltiorrhizae (*Dan Shen*)	15 grams
Radix Polygoni Multiflori (*He Shou Wu*)	15 grams
Radix Glehniae Littoralis (*Bei Sha Shen*)	15 grams

Method of administration: Place these herbs in a pot with 1,000ml of water and boil until 800ml of liquid is left. Use 1 packet per day, dividing the herbal tea into 3-4 portions drunk throughout the day. White sugar may be added to sweeten the tea. These herbs may also be stewed for soup. Drink the soup as a tea.

Functions: Supplements the kidneys and nourishes the stomach, engenders fluids and replenishes the essence, quickens the blood and frees the vessels, retards aging and dispels disease

Indications: This tea is suitable for the treatment of lung/kidney yin vacuity with static blood. It has the special effect of quickening the blood, nourishing the heart, and reducing weight in middle-aged and elderly individuals with high cholesterol and increased blood viscosity.

Five Fragrance Milk Tea (*Wu Xiang Nai Cha*)

Cow's milk (*Niu Nai*)	A suitable amount
Tea leaves, *i.e.*, Folium Camelliae Theae (*Cha Ye*)	A suitable amount
White sugar (*Bai Tang*)	A suitable amount
Honey (*Feng Mi*)	A suitable amount
Almond (*Tian Xing Ren*)	A suitable amount
Sesame seed, *i.e.,* Semen Sesami Indici (*Zhi Ma*)	A suitable amount

Method of administration: Grind the almonds and sesame into a fine powder. Add the Tea leaves to the milk and boil, to make milk Tea. Then add the almond and sesame powder to this milk Tea. One should also add honey and/or white sugar. This may be taken as a breakfast or snack food.

Functions: Supplements the spleen and kidneys and benefits longevity

Indications: This tea is suitable for the treatment of malnutrition, a weak constitution, and premature senility.

Old Age Protect the Health Tea (*Lao Nian Bao Jian Cha*)

Polished, round-grained, non-glutinous rice, *i.e.*, Semen Oryzae Sativae (*Jing Mi*)	60 grams
Deep-fried walnut, *i.e.*, deep-fried Semen Juglandis Regiae (*You Zhi Hu Tao Rou*)	60 grams
Uncooked walnut, *i.e.*, uncooked Semen Juglandis Regiae (*Sheng Hu Tao Rou*)	50 grams
Cow's milk (*Niu Nai*)	200 grams
White sugar (*Bai Tang*)	Amount to taste

Method of administration: Rinse the rice well and let it soak for 1 hour. Scoop up the rice and filter out the soaking water. Mix the rice with the two kinds of walnuts and the milk, grinding this mixture into a thick liquid. Filter and save the liquid. Add sugar to some boiled water. Then pour in the filtered liquid. Stir this evenly while pouring and bring it to another boil. Drink the resulting liquid as a tea, 1-2 times per day.

Functions: Fortifies the spleen and boosts the qi, supplements the blood and moistens dryness, expels stones

Indications: This tea is suitable for the treatment of dry intestines constipation and stone strangury. It can also be used as a health protection drink that moistens the skin and blackens the hair, invigorates yang and secures the essence. Taken often, this formula can regulate the metabolism of the aging body, prolong life, and benefit longevity.

Contraindications: This formula is warming. Therefore, individuals with phlegm fire symptoms, such as coughing up yellow, sticky phlegm, a dry mouth and throat, and a thick, yellow tongue coating, should not use this formula.

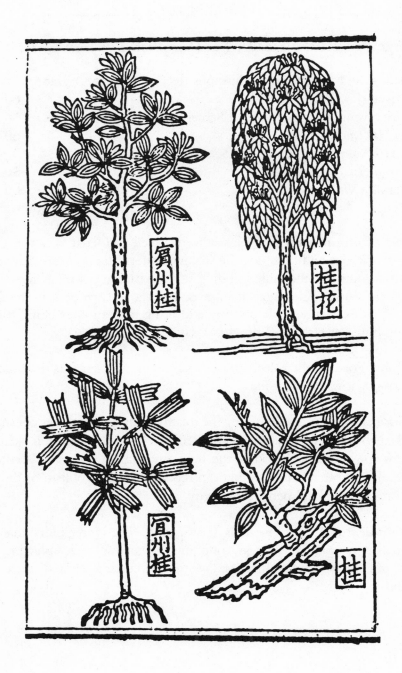

賓州桂

桂花

宜州桂

桂

16
Getting Started

Where to get the ingredients

In order to make use of the various Chinese medicinal tea formulas in this book, one must be able to either find or purchase the ingredients. As stated in the introduction, those ingredients whose names first appear in common English are either available in grocery, health food, or Oriental specialty food stores or can be found growing locally. Those ingredients whose names are given in Latin and Pinyin only must be ordered from Chinese herbal suppliers. The following list of Chinese herbal suppliers all sell Chinese herbs through the mail.

In the United States of America:

Spring Wind Herb Company
2315 Fourth St.
Berkeley, CA 94710
Tel. 510-849-1820
Fax: 510-849-4886
Orders: 1-800-588-4883

(The above company goes to great lengths to import and sell Chinese herbs free from pesticides, fungicides, bleaches, and other chemical contaminants.)

China Herb Co.
165 W. Queen Lane
Philadelphia, PA 19144
Tel. 215-843-5864
Fax: 215-849-3338
Orders: 1-800-221-4372

Nuherbs Co.
3820 Penniman Ave.
Oakland, CA 94619
Tel. 415-534-4372
Orders: 1-800-233-4307

In the United Kingdom:

Acumedic Ltd.
101-105 Camden High Street
London NW1 7JN
Tel. 0171-3886704
Fax: 0171-3875766

East West Herb Shop
3 Neals Yard
Covent Garden, London WC2H 9DP
Tel. 0171-3791312
Fax: 0171-3794414

East West Herbs Ltd.
Langston Priory Mews
Kingham, Oxfordshire OX7 6UP
Tel. 01608-658862
Fax: 01608-658816

Harmony Acupuncture
Supplies Center
629 High Road Leytonstone
London E11 4PA
Tel. 0181-518-7337
Fax: 0181-518-7338

Mayway Herbal Emporium
43 Waterside Trading Estate
Trumpers Way, Hanwell,
London W7
Tel. 0181-459-1812
Fax: 0181-459-1727

In Europe:

Belgium
Tai Yang Chinese Herb Store
Poperingseweg 271
8908 Vlamertinge
Ieper
Tel. 057-21-86-69
Fax: 057-21-97-78

China's Nature N.V.
Huyslaan 37
B-8790 Waregem
Tel: 32 (0)56 603307
Fax: 32 (0)56 612907

Homeofar
Hugo Verriestlaan 63
8500 Kortrijk
Tel: 32-56-22-8916
Fax: 32-56-22-7113

Sinecura
Krijglaan 151
9000 Gent
Tel: 32-9-244-6868
Fax: 32-9-244-6849

Ireland
P.P.C. Ltd.
Tel. 091-753-222
Fax: 091-753-471

Denmark
Dragon Herbs
Tel. 44-66-21-14
Fax: 44-66-21-15

Netherlands
Euroherbs
Claassenland 15
NL-6932 AZ
Westervoort
Tel. O8-303-15660
Fax: 08-303-17752

Chinese Medical Center
Geldersekade 67-73
1011 EK Amsterdam
Tel. 31 020-623-50-60
Fax: 31 020-623-36-36

Italy
East West Herbs
Tel. 06-90-66-813
Fax: 06-90-66-813

Spain
East West Herbs
Tel. 1-539-0862
Fax: 1-639-0862

Portugal
East West Herbs
Tel. 1-486-4356
Fax: 1-486-4556

France
Harmonia I Naturalesa
L'Artisan Herboriste
BP 117
Andorra La Vella
ANDORA, via France
Tel: 33-376-835-566

In Australia:

Chinaherb
82-84 George St.
Refern Syndney 2016
Tel. 02-698-5555 (Sydney area)
Tel. 1800 024-286
(outside Sydney)
Tel. 07-369-0045 (Queensland)
Fax: 02-698-5755

Where to find out more about Chinese herbal medicine

In order to select the right Chinese medicinal tea for the right person, it is important to have a basic understanding of each medicinal's properties, functions, indications, and contraindications. The ingredients in this book are basically divided into two broad categories: herbs and foods. For information on the medicinal properties, functions, and indications of Chinese medicinal herbs, the reader should see Dan Bensky & Andrew Gamble's *Chinese Herbal Medicine: Materia Medica* published by Eastland Press. For information on the Chinese medicinal properties, functions, and indications of Chinese medicinal foods, the reader is recommended to Bob Flaws & Honora Lee Wolfe's *Prince Wen Hui's Cook: Chinese Dietary Therapy* published by Paradigm Publications.

In addition and as explained in the Introduction, TCM bases its treatment on pattern discrimination and not just upon the patient's named disease or main symptom. Therefore, the more one understands about TCM pattern discrimination, the better one will be able to match up the formulas in this book to individual persons. For more information on TCM pattern discrimination, the reader should see Ted Kaptchuk's *The Web That Has No Weaver: Understanding Chinese Medicine* published by Congdon & Weed. This is the single best introduction to TCM and does include the signs and symptoms, including tongue and pulse signs, of all the main TCM patterns. Another book specifically about distinguishing TCM patterns is Bob Flaws & Daniel Finney's *A Compendium of TCM Patterns & Treatments* published by Blue Poppy Press.

In some instances, the formulas in this book specify that a particular ingredient is supposed to be processed in some manner before being used according to the directions in this book. For instance, some herbs are to be stir-fried, while others should be mix-fried. Some shoud be earth stir-fried, and yet others should be scorched or roasted. In Chinese medicine, the processing of Chinese herbs before they are used in a prescription is a science all of its own. Depending on how an ingredient is processed, it changes that ingredient's nature and indications. For more information on this science of processing Chinese herbs prior to use, the reader should see Philippe Sionneau's *Pao Zhi: An Introduction to the Use of Processed Chinese Medicinals* published by Blue Poppy Press.

And finally, if you have enjoyed this book on Chinese medicinal teas, you would probably also enjoy two other Blue Poppy Press books. These are *Chinese Medicinal Wines & Elixirs* and *The Book of Jook: Chinese Medicinal Porridges* both by Bob Flaws.

How to find a TCM practitioner

For those lay readers who would like to make use of the information in this book, the authors and publishers highly recommend seeing a well-trained and experienced, professional practitioner of Chinese medicine in order to get an accurate TCM pattern discrimination and to select the right medicinal tea. Because most such professional practitioners of TCM are legally permitted to practice under various acupuncture licensing laws (at least in the U.S.), the reader should look in their Yellow Pages under the heading Acupuncturists. In the U.S., there is a National Commission for the Certification of Acupuncturists (NCCA). This commission certifies practitioners in both acupuncture specifically and in Chinese herbal medicine. In order to become certified, practitioners have to have graduated from approved schools with a minimum number of hours of training *and* they must have passed a comprehensive examination. Practitioners who are NCCA certified in Chinese herbal medicine append the letters Dipl. C.H. after their names. This stands for Diplomate of Chinese Herbs. We highly recommend our readers to seek out such NCCA diplomates when seeking a TCM pattern discrimination and advice on Chinese medicinal teas. The NCCA does supply information on its diplomates in local areas. They can be reached at:

The National Commission for the Certification of Acupuncturists
1424 16th St. NW, Suite 501
Washington, DC 20036
Tel. 202-232-1404, Fax: 202-462-6157

In the United States there are also two large national professional associations of acupuncturists and Chinese medical practitioners. These associations can also supply the names and addresses of their members in local areas:

National Acupuncture & Oriental Medicine Alliance
P.O. Box 77511
Seattle, WA 98177-0531
Tel. 206-524-3511, Fax: 206-728-4841,
e-mail: 76143.2061@compuserve.com

American Association of Acupuncture & Oriental Medicine
433 Front St.
Catasauqua, PA 18032-2506
Tel. 610-433-2448, Fax: 610-433-1832

In addition, in states where the independent practice of acupuncture is legal, either the State Department of Health or the Department of Regulatory Agencies can furnish a list of all licensed acupuncturists within that state. These agencies cannot tell you who is good or bad or who has been trained in what, but they can usually give you the addresses and telephone numbers of state professional associations. These state professional associations typically are able to make local referrals which are based on training, experience, and style of practice.

Another possibility for finding a local practitioner in the U.S. is to contact:

The National Accreditation Commission for Schools & Colleges of Acupuncture and Oriental Medicine
1010 Wayne Ave., Suite 1270
Silver Springs, MD 20910
Tel. 301-608-9680, Fax: 301-608-9576

This commission acredits schools and colleges of acupuncture and Oriental medicine in the U.S. They can give you the names and addresses of such schools in local areas. Then, by calling one of the schools in your area, the school can give you the names and addresses of graduates practicing in that area. In general, schools which are accredited have better curricula and higher standards than nonaccredited schools, and, therefore, their graduates are often better trained and more knowledgable than graduates of other schools.

In areas where acupuncture and Oriental medicine are not legally recognized independent professions, one can usually find local practitioners by asking at neighborhood health food stores. Clerks at health food stores typically hear from their customers who practices what locally and who the good practitioners are. Word of mouth from satisfied customers is always an important factor when considering a health care provider. Further, when interviewing a potential Chinese medical practitioner, we believe that you should ask where they were trained, for how long, and are they specifically trained in Chinese herbal medicine. Some practitioners are only acupuncturists and have not been formally trained in Chinese herbal medicine.

How to tell if a medicinal tea is working

Sometimes it is hard at first for the layperson to tell if a Chinese medicinal tea is working or not. If a person drinks a couple of doses of a medicinal tea and all their symptoms completely disappear, then it is pretty obvious that the tea is beneficial. But it does not always happen that way and especially not for chronic diseases with long-standing or recurrent symptoms.

There are six key questions you can ask yourself to help determine if a Chinese medicinal tea is good for you or not, after having taken it for a while. These questions are:

1. How is my digestion?
2. How are my bowel movements?
3. How is my appetite?

4. How is my sleep?
5. How is my energy?
6. How is my mood?

If the answer to these six questions is that all these areas are better than they were, then it is pretty sure that the medicinal tea is doing you some real good. However, if after taking the medicinal tea for a few days, one or more of these areas has gotten worse, then that tea is not perfectly matched to you and your pattern. It may be that some of these six areas get better and one or two get worse. In that case, the situation is mixed. Although the tea is doing some good, there are negative side effects. Since Chinese medicine works by achieving balance in the entire body, Chinese doctors believe that the only real healing is healing without side effects. Therefore, if a Chinese herbal tea causes any of the above six areas to get worse than they were before starting the tea, the tea should be discontinued and professional advice sought. If the tea is correctly matched to the person's TCM pattern of disharmony, than all six of these basic parameters of health should take a turn for the better.

Conclusion

Traditional Chinese medicine is the oldest, continually practiced, literate, professional medicine in the world. The wisdom of Chinese medicine has been honed for over more than a hundred generations of professional practitioners who have recorded their experiences in each generation in tens of thousands of books which still survive to this day. Because of its efficacy and freedom from side effects, TCM has been selected by the World Health Organization (WHO) for worldwide propagation in the 21st century. The Chinese medicinal teas contained in this book are part of the accumulated medical wisdom of the Chinese people and are a very simple and easy way for Westerners to begin experiencing for themselves the healing benefits of this ancient health care system.

Bibliography

Chinese language bibliography

Ben Cao Gang Mu (The Detailed Outline of the Materia Medica), Li Shi-zhen, Ming dynasty, People's Health & Hygiene Press, Beijing, 1985

Da Zhong Yao Shan (Medicinal Meals of the Masses), Peng Ming-quan, Sichuan Science & Technology Press, Chengdu, 1985

Han Ying Chang Yong Yi Xue Ci Hui (A Chinese-English Collection of Commonly Used Medical Words), People's Health & Hygiene Press, Beijing, 1982

Han Ying Yi Xue Da Ci Dian (Chinese-English Medical Dictionary), People's Health & Hygiene Press, Beijing, 1988

Jia Ting Yao Cha (Family Medicinal Teas), Wang Fa-wei & Hao Ai-zhen, Whole Shield Press, Beijing, 1993

Min Jian Pian Fang Mi Fang Jing Xuan (An Essential Collection of Folk & Secret Formulas of the People), Zheng Qing-liang, People's Army Medical Press, Beijing, 1990

Pian Fang Da Quan (A Great Collection of Folk Formulas), Beijing Science & Technology Press, Beijing, 1990

Pu Ji Fang (Universal Benefit Formulas), Zhu Ti, Ming dynasty, People's Health & Hygiene Press, Beijing, 1982

Qian Shi Shi Zhi (Food Treatments [from the Prescriptions Worth a] Thousand [Pieces of] Gold), Sun Si-miao, Tang Dynasty; *Shi Liao Fang (Food Treatment Formulas)*, Hu Si-hui, Yuan dynasty, Commercial Press of China, Beijing, 1985

Quan Guo Zhong Cao Yao Hui Bian (All National Chinese Herbal Medicinals Collection), People's Health & Hygiene Press, Beijing, 1986

Shi Wu Zhong Yao Yu Bian Fang (Foodstuff Chinese Medicinal Adjunctive Formulas), Ye Ku-quan, Jiangsu Science & Technology Press, Nanjing, 1980

Shi Zhi Ben Cao (A Materia Medica of Dietary Therapy), Jiang Qing-yun, Earth Wisdom Press, Beijing, 1990

Tai Ping Sheng Hui Fang (Tai Ping Imperial Grace Formulary), Wang Huai-yin, Song dynasty, People's Health & Hygiene Press, Beijing, 1982

Yin Shi Liao Fa (Food & Drink Therapy), Hu Hai-tian & Liang Jian-hui, Guandong Technical Press, Guangzhou, 1987

Zhong Hua Shi Wu Liao Fa Da Quan (A Great Collection of Foodstuff Treatments from China), Dou Guo-xiang, Jiangsu Science & Technology Press, Taizhou, 1990

Zhong Yao Bie Ming Shou Ce (A Handbook of Chinese Medicinal Alternative Names), Bao Xi-sheng, Guandong Science & Technology Press, Guangzhou, 1993

English language bibliography

A Compendium of TCM Patterns & Treatments, Bob Flaws & Daniel Finney, Blue Poppy Press, Boulder, CO, 1996

An Enumeration of Chinese Materia Medica, Shui-ying Hu, The Chinese University Press, Hong Kong, 1980

Arisal of the Clear: A Simple Guide to Healthy Eating According to Traditional Chinese Medicine, Bob Flaws, Blue Poppy Press, Boulder, CO, 1991

Basic Theory of Traditional Chinese Medicine, Vol. 1 & 2, Zhang En-qin, ed., Shanghai College of Chinese Medicine Press, Shanghai, 1991

Chinese-English Medical Dictionary, Cui Yue Li, ed., Business & Commerce Publications, Hong Kong, 1988

Chinese Herbal Medicine: Formulas & Strategies, Dan Bensky & Randall Barolet, Eastland Press, Seattle, WA, 1990

Chinese Herbal Medicine: Materia Medica, Dan Bensky & Andrew Gamble, Eastland Press, Seattle, WA, 1986

Chinese Herbal Remedies, Albert Y. Leung, Universe Books, NY, 1984

Chinese Medicated Diet, Zhang En-qin, ed., Shanghai College of Chinese Medicine Press, Shanghai, 1991

Chinese Medicinal Wines & Elixirs, Bob Flaws, Blue Poppy Press, Boulder, CO, 1994

Chinese System of Food Cures: Prevention & Remedies, Henry C. Lu, Sterling Publishing Co., NY, 1986

Eating Your Way to Healthy: Dietotherapy in Traditional Chinese Medicine, Cai Jing-feng, Foreign Languages Press, Beijing, 1988

English-Chinese Chinese-English Dictionary of Chinese Medicine, Nigel Wiseman, Hunan Science & Technology Press, Changsha, 1995

English-Chinese Medical Dictionary, People's Health & Hygiene Press, Beijing, 1995

Fruit as Medicine, Dai Yin-fang & Liu Cheng-jun, trans. by Ron Edwards & Gong Zhi-mei, The Rams Skull Press, Kuranda, Australia, 1987

Fundamentals of Chinese Medicine, East Asian Medical Studies Society, Paradigm Publications, Brookline, MA, 1985

Glossary of Chinese Medical Terms and Acupuncture Points, Nigel Wiseman *et al.*, Paradigm Publications, Brookline, MA, 1990

Harmony Rules: The Chinese Way of Health Through Food, Gary Butt & Frena Bloomfield, Samuel Weiser Inc., York Beach, ME, 1987

Imperial Secrets of Health & Longevity, Bob Flaws, Blue Poppy Press, Boulder, CO, 1994

Legendary Chinese Healing Herbs, Henry C. Lu, Sterling Publishing Co., NY, 1991

Oriental Materia Medica: A Concise Guide, Hong-yen Hsu *et al.,* Oriental Healing Arts Insitute, Long Beach, CA, 1986

Pao Zhi: An Introduction to the Use of Processed Chinese Medicinals, Philippe Sionneau, Blue Poppy Press, Boulder, CO, 1995

Prince Wen Hui's Cook: Chinese Dietary Therapy, Bob Flaws & Honora Lee Wolfe, Paradigm Publications, Brookline, MA, 1983

Tabers Cyclopedic Medicinal Dictionary, Clayton Thomas , ed. , Davis Company, Philadelphia, PA, 1979

The Book of Jook: Chinese Medicinal Porridges, Bob Flaws, Blue Poppy Press, Boulder, CO, 1995

The English-Chinese Encyclopedia of Practical Traditional Chinese Medicine: Simple and Proven Recipes, Xu Xiang-cai, ed., Higher Education Press, Beijing, 1991

The Illustrated Chinese Materia Medica: *Crude and Prepared*, Kun-Ying Yen, SMC Publishing, Taipei, Taiwan, 1992

The Tao of Nutrition, Maoshing Ni & Cathy McNease, The Shrine of the Eternal Breath of Tao, Malibu, CA, 1987

The Web That Has No Weaver: Understanding Chinese Medicine, Ted Kaptchuk, Congdon & Weed, NY, 1983

Traditional Medicine in Contemporary China, Nathan Sivin, Center for Chinese Studies, Univ. of Michigan, Ann Arbor, MI, 1987

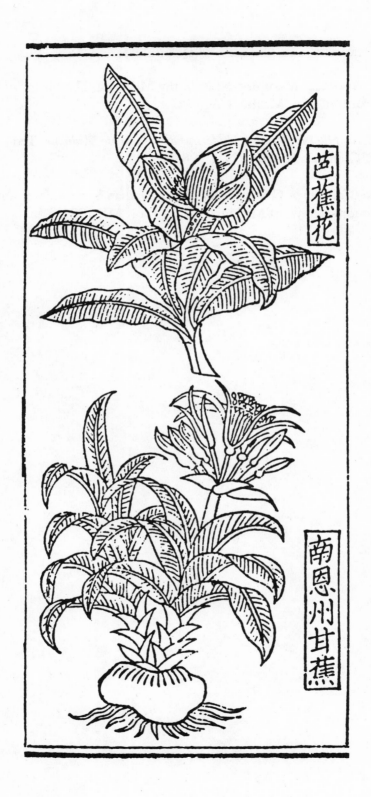

芭蕉花

南恩州甘蕉

Index

A

A Discussion of the Medical Formulas of Ci Xi & Guang Xu 11
abdomen, aching and pain within the 46
abdomen, distention and pain in the lower 164
abdomen, downward sagging feeling in the 249
abdomen, dull pain in the lower 163
abdominal chilly or gripping pain, lower 166
abdominal cramping 250
abdominal distention 13, 14, 38, 43, 63, 165, 200, 222, 280
abdominal pain 20, 29, 43, 44, 49, 57, 127, 160, 163, 165, 166, 171, 172, 176, 201, 251, 272, 274, 279
abdominal pain during pregnancy, lower 172
abdominal pain, intolerable 127
abdominal pain, postpartum 160, 165, 176
acid regurgitation 38
alcohol toxins 128, 257
allergic rhinitis 214
amenorrhea 159, 165, 167, 266
angina pectoris 92, 93
angiocardiopathy 93, 98
aphasia 98
appetite, loss of 36
Arisal of the Clear: A Simple Guide to Healthy Eating According to Chinese Medicine 9
arteriosclerosis 119, 284
ascites 63-65, 209, 248
asthma 25, 27, 29

B

bee stings 138
belching 31, 35, 38, 106, 227
belching of putrid gas 38
Ben Cao Gang Mu 11
bi syndrome 99
biliary ascariasis 127
bladder, cancer of the 245, 251
bladder stones 79
bleeding, spontaneous external 43, 220
bleeding, sudden onset of 161
blindness, night 211, 212
blood flukes 63

blood pressure, high 72, 85, 90
blood pressure, low 89, 91, 271
bodily heaviness 231
body and limbs, cold 274
body, hot 57
body pain 15, 16, 18
body, thin, with lack of strength 140
bone and joint pain 101
bones, pain in the sinews and 102
Book of Jook: Chinese Medicinal Porridges 9, 296
borborygmus 31, 249
breast cancer 247, 253, 254
breast *yong* 180, 181
breath, bad 37, 198, 199, 227
breathing with an open mouth 30
brightness, shying away from 207, 208, 212
bronchial asthma 27
bronchitis 22, 25-27, 190
Buerger's disease 98

C

Camellia Thea 10
canker sores 216
carbuncles and sores 19
carcinoma of the liver 247, 248
cardiac murmur 93
cardiovascular diseases 85
cataracts 212
cerebral embolism 97
cerebral hemorrhage 97
cerebral thrombosis 97, 98
cerebral vascular accident 97
cerebrovascular spasm 97
cheek, mild swelling of the 18
cheeks, flushed red 35
chest and epigastrium, glomus and oppression in the 242
chest oppression 20, 35, 91, 94, 116, 123, 227, 238, 261
chest pain 43, 106, 236
chest, pain in the, and lateral costal regions 106
chest, vexation and oppression within the 39
chickenpox 196, 197
Chinese Medicinal Wines & Elixirs 9, 153, 296
chloasma 143
cholecystitis 69-72

OTHER BOOKS ON CHINESE MEDICINE FROM BLUE POPPY PRESS

3450 Penrose Place, Suite 110, Boulder, CO 80301
For ordering 1-800-487-9296 PH. 303\447-8372 FAX 303\245-8362

A NEW AMERICAN ACUPUNCTURE

ACUPOINT POCKET REFERENCE

ACUPUNCTURE AND MOXIBUSTION FORMULAS & TREATMENTS

ACUTE ABDOMINAL SYNDROMES

AGING & BLOOD STASIS: A New Approach to TCM Geriatrics

AIDS & ITS TREATMENT IN TCM

BETTER BREAST HEALTH NATURALLY with CHINESE MEDICINE

THE BOOK OF JOOK: Chinese Medicinal Porridges

CHINESE MEDICAL PALMISTRY: Your Health in Your Hand

CHINESE MEDICINAL TEAS: Simple, Proven, Folk Formulas for Common Diseases & Promoting Health

CHINESE MEDICINAL WINES & ELIXIRS

CHINESE PEDIATRIC MASSAGE THERAPY: *A Parent's & Practitioner's Guide*

CHINESE SELF-MASSAGE THERAPY: The Easy Way to Health

A COMPENDIUM OF TCM PATTERNS & TREATMENTS

CURING ARTHRITIS NATURALLY WITH CHINESE MEDICINE

CURING DEPRESSION NATURALLY WITH CHINESE MEDICINE

CURING HAY FEVER NATURALLY WITH CHINESE MEDICINE

CURING HEADACHES NATURALLY WITH CHINESE MEDICINE

CURING INSOMNIA NATURALLY WITH CHINESE MEDICINE

CURING PMS NATURALLY WITH CHINESE MEDICINE

THE DAO OF INCREASING LONGEVITY & CONSERVING ONE'S LIFE

A STUDY OF DAOIST ACUPUNCTURE & MOXIBUSTION

THE DIVINE FARMER'S MATERIA MEDICA

THE DIVINELY RESPONDING CLASSIC: *A Translation of the Shen Ying Jing*

DUI YAO: THE ART OF COMBINING CHINESE HERBAL MEDICINALS

ENDOMETRIOSIS, INFERTILITY AND TRADITIONAL CHINESE MEDICINE

THE ESSENCE OF LIU FENG-WU'S GYNECOLOGY

EXTRA TREATISES BASED ON INVESTIGATION & INQUIRY

FIRE IN THE VALLEY: TCM Diagnosis & Treatment of Vaginal Diseases

FU QING-ZHU'S GYNECOLOGY

FULFILLING THE ESSENCE: A *Handbook of Traditional & Contemporary Treatments for Female Infertility*

GOLDEN NEEDLE WANG LE-TING: A 20th Century Master's Approach to Acupuncture

A HANDBOOK OF TRADITIONAL CHINESE DERMATOLOGY

A HANDBOOK OF TRADITIONAL CHINESE GYNECOLOGY

A HANDBOOK OF MENSTRUAL DISEASES IN CHINESE MEDICINE